THE FALLING SHADOW

Publication Statement, 16 January 1995

Louis Blom-Cooper, Helen Hally and Elaine Murphy

Our advocacy in the final chapter of *The Falling Shadow* for an official review of mental health legislation, with a view to replacing the *obsolescent* Mental Health Act 1983 – a word used by the House of Commons Select Committee for Health in its recent report – was no act of whimsy on our part. It may be said, with some justification, that the deficiencies exposed in our report on the policies and practices of the South Devon Healthcare Trust could and should have been avoided by the managers and practitioners performing their tasks properly within the existing legal framework for mental health. But, however, our view that much of the maladministration and malpractices derived from a fundamentally flawed statutory framework. A different legislative approach would have produced different practices and better results. Our final chapter, which is devoted exclusively to an argument for an entirely new approach to the care and treatment of the mentally disordered, deliberately does not relate to the events and occurrences examined throughout the report. It could usefully have done so. We now proceed to do just that in this epilogue to the report.

The first flaw is the Act's underlying theme that care and treatment for people with mental disorder of a certain severity can be provided only by detention in hospital. The place where care and treatment is delivered – the hospital – without the patient's consent is inseparable in the 1983 Act from a place of residence for detention. Had that underlying theme not been so dominant in psychiatric thinking, practitioners would not have been so reluctant to use their powers to detain Andrew Robinson, or at least not delayed the exercise of their powers of compulsory admission. The faulty interpretation of those powers, which we have exposed in Chapter XVIII (Admission under the Mental Health Act 1983), would never have been adopted psychiatrically in Andrew Robinson's case, to his detriment, had there not been such an emphasis on the civil liberties of the mentally ill.

The philosophy of the 1983 Act focuses on society's intervention in curtailing the liberty of the individual. It fails to make any philosophical statement of the nature of the liberty of the mentally unwell patient. Had it done so, the legislative message to all professional carers, and not just those involved in the immediate process of compulsory admission – the registered medical practitioners and the approved social workers – would have induced a more effective multi-disciplinary approach to Andrew Robinson's case. Moreover, the removal by the Mental Health Review Tribunal in September 1986 of the power to recall Andrew Robinson (related in Chapter IX) would not have happened if there had been a multi-disciplinary ingredient in the Tribunal's decision, instead of a total reliance on the opinion of Andrew Robinson's RMO. Even if one might expect a better result from a tribunal sitting to hear Andrew Robinson's case in 1995, there are sufficient worries about the working of Mental Health Review Tribunals to warrant an urgent review. The Council on Tribunals, the watchdog body for all administrative tribunals, has voiced in its last two Annual Reports its concern about certain aspects of the procedures of MHRTs.

The second fundamental flaw that afflicted the actions and omissions of the professional carers of Andrew Robinson was the dissociation of psychiatric treatment from the social context in which care must be delivered in order to be therapeutic. The 1983 Act is a means of facilitating but controlling the specific health care interventions of doctors in the lives of mentally ill people. It focuses not on patients, but on doctors. Thus the non-continuance in Andrew Robinson's case of the Guardianship Order beyond July 1992 was prompted precisely because the authors of it viewed the impact of the Order from a medical stand-point, and not with the ongoing need for supervised care in mind. Legislation grounded in a community care approach would have propelled the practitioners, and not just gently prompted them (as we indicate in Chapter IX that they ought to have been prompted) to keep the Guardianship Order in being indefinitely.

Until the mental health legislation is turned upside down – admission to an institution, whether compulsory or voluntary, being given a secondary role in care and treatment – practitioners will continue to view their powers and responsibilities as institutionally based rather than community focused. Once Andrew Robinson was discharged conditionally from Broadmoor in 1981, the residual liability to recall should have remained as a last resort for continuous community care. The seven successive admissions to the Edith Morgan Centre from 1986 to 1993 were part and parcel of a philosophy directed, if not dictated, by outmoded mental health legislation.

THE FALLING SHADOW

One patient's mental health care
1978-1993

Report of the Committee of Inquiry into the events
leading up to and surrounding the fatal incident at the
Edith Morgan Centre, Torbay, on 1 September 1993*

*Louis Blom-Cooper
Helen Hally
Elaine Murphy

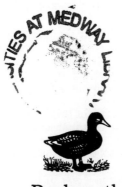

Duckworth

Between the desire
And the spasm
Between the potency
And the existence
Between the essence
And the descent
Falls the Shadow

T.S. Eliot,
The Hollow Men
(1926)

This impression 2001
First published in 1995 by
Gerald Duckworth & Co. Ltd.
61 Frith Street, London W1D 3JL
Tel: 020 7434 4242
Fax: 020 7434 4420
Email: inquiries@duckworth-publishers.co.uk
www.ducknet.co.uk

A catalogue record for this book is available
from the British Library

ISBN 0 7156 2662 0

Printed in Great Britain by
Antony Rowe Ltd, Eastbourne

Contents

Part D. General Issues

Appendices

Acknowledgments

No public inquiry can hope to achieve the desired twin objectives of thoroughness and fairness without a thorough preparation, well in advance of the oral hearings. All the relevant documentation needs to be painstakingly retrieved from the files of organisations and individuals involved. Only after that documentation has been assembled, sifted for its materiality and organised to meet the needs of the inquiry team, is it sensible to approach prospective witnesses for written statements. Either because of the sheer size of the task – often the documentation is voluminous and not always well- arranged – or because the inquiry team wishes to preserve the semblance of impartiality, the team needs professional assistance in ingesting and digesting the material. In short, any public inquiry demands from the outset the active participation of counsel.

Our appointment of Mr Oliver Thorold and Ms Michelle Strange as counsel to the Inquiry was indispensable. With the indefatigable administrative assistance of Mrs Jackie Barrett at the headquarters of the South Devon Healthcare Trust in Torbay, they collected all the documentation and prepared, progressively through five editions, a chronology of events (infinitely longer than the one we include here for the reader who wants a quick and easy reference). The chronology not only provided us with an early picture of the main issues that were likely to arise from our detailed consideration, but was also crucial to the prospective witnesses. Because of the need to cover events ranging over at least a decade, it was inevitable that many of the actors in the events could not remember exactly what happened. The chronology jogged many a memory. The letters which went out to prospective witnesses invariably included the chronology, with cross-reference to the specific questions which the witnesses were asked to address. This exercise hugely facilitated the process of the Inquiry and undoubtedly shortened the oral hearings, both in limiting the number of witnesses and in reducing the length of time needed to canvass further the matters to which the witnesses had alluded (or omitted to allude) in their written statements. The value of the chronology lay not merely in the simple exercise of putting a happening to a date in chronological order. The manner in which the Thorold/Strange chronology was carried out was a model of pinpointing significant events, highlighting shifts in the care and treatment of Andrew Robinson, and in indicating the issues for us to tackle. Their assimilation of the massive evidence became impressively evident when they conducted the questioning of the witnesses. Our gratitude to them is boundless.

The only other lawyers engaged in the Inquiry were Ms Nichola Davies, assisted by junior counsel and a solicitor from Bevan Ashford, solicitors to the Trust. Their participation in the Inquiry was never less than helpful. Since most of the witnesses were or still are employees of South Devon Healthcare Trust, Ms Davies led the questioning of them. She was always economical in her questions and assisted materially in advancing the cause of an efficient and effective inquiry, while maintaining a proper regard for her clients' interests. We received a written memorandum from Ms Davies on 9 November 1994, in time for us to take on board all the submissions which she made on behalf of the Trust and the Trust's witnesses.

Throughout the Inquiry we have had the invaluable assistance of Dr John Crichton, Nightingale Research Scholar and Honorary Registrar in Psychiatry, University of Cambridge, Institute of Criminology. We invited him, in particular, to organise the one-day seminar on 1 August 1994 at the conclusion of the oral hearings – also held in public. His introductory paper reviewing the current literature concerning psychiatric inpatient violence and commentary on contemporary knowledge about the prediction of violent behaviour of the mentally disordered was an excellent piece of work. It greatly informed the two topics of the seminar. Dr Crichton also undertook all the arrangements for obtaining the speakers at the seminar and for preparing their papers for a book, *Psychiatric Patient Violence*, which is published simultaneously with this report. We are enormously grateful to him also for assisting us with some knotty psychiatric problems that cropped up during the Inquiry.

Our thanks for facilitating the Inquiry go to the South Devon Healthcare Trust. Its readiness to set up the Inquiry and allow us full rein to conduct it in public in our own manner has been very welcome. The Chairman, Mr Tony Boyce OBE, was particularly supportive of our efforts to hold the Inquiry free from any improper interference. The Trust's Chief Executive, Mr Tony Parr, likewise responded to all our calls for administrative assistance. The facilities at the Old Forde House in Newton Abbot (the administrative building of the local authority) admirably suited our requirements for relaxed informality in pleasant surroundings. On the final day of the hearing, which was held at the educational unit of the hospital, Georgina Robinson's family expressed their distress at being brought back to the site where their daughter died. We apologised to the Robinsons at the time – the decision to move the venue of the Inquiry from Newton Abbot to Torbay Hospital had been entirely ours – and we repeat our regrets at a lapse in our sensitivity to their plight. Elsewhere (Chapter I) we have paid tribute to both Robinson families for the dignified and restrained manner in which they conducted themselves during a period which brought back the unhappiest of times in their recent lives.

Finally, we should like to thank all those who participated in the Inquiry, too many to name. Being subjected retrospectively (often going back many years) to minute scrutiny of one's actions can be disconcerting. To have to undergo such examination under the public spotlight of media attention and press and TV coverage is certainly painful. But we do not apologise for having over-ridden a wish, expressed informally, for rather less publicity. Those who provide a public service must accept that they are publicly accountable for their work. And that means accounting for their actions in a public forum.

At our oral hearings the burdensome task of organising the witnesses and making the manifold administrative arrangements was performed with consummate ease by Mrs Jackie Barrett and, for the first of the two weeks, Mr Alex Bax. Their assiduity greatly eased our ability to pay undivided and undeflected attention to the witnesses' evidence.

Last, but decidedly not least, our thanks are due to Chris Thomas who was unpardonably deflected from her secretarial duties to one of us (EM). She was uncomplaining in translating our manuscript drafts – from one of us (not to be publicly identified) in execrable handwriting – onto the word processor. That we have managed to keep to a rigorous timetable is due almost entirely to the speed and efficiency with which she turned our scribblings into a manuscript for the publishers. We were delighted that the Trust agreed to our suggestion that Gerald Duckworth & Co should publish our report, together with the papers delivered at the seminar. It was an immense sadness that Duckworth's managing director, Mr Colin Haycraft, died suddenly on 24 September 1994.

Dramatis Personae

In order to have a full and easy understanding of the events under inquiry, and of the individuals involved in the events, the reader of this report needs to know something about the occupations and posts held by those who participated. Rather than interpose such particulars in the course of this lengthy and unavoidably discursive account, we have included a list of them here. This will avoid the need to identify named persons at any point in the text.

Victim of assault, 1 September 1993

Georgina Robinson, born 30 September 1966, Occupational Therapist, Edith Morgan Centre, 1991-1993. Died 7 October 1993.

Patient

Andrew Ross Robinson, born 28 November 1957, found guilty of manslaughter of Georgina Robinson (no relation) at Truro Crown Court on 22 March 1994; committed to Broadmoor Hospital under Section 37/41 of the Mental Health Act 1983.

Families

Gordon Brian Robinson and (Florence) Wendy Robinson, parents of Georgina Robinson.

Reverend (retired) Peter McCall Robinson and Jennifer Patricia Robinson, parents of Andrew Robinson.

Doctors

Dr S. Cannizarro, SHO to Dr Moss, November 1989.

Dr Gerald Conway, retired (since March 1991) consultant psychiatrist. RMO to Andrew Robinson in the community and at Moorhaven Hospital from 1982-1986.

Dr Moira (Molly) Cullen, working in public health, Wirral Health Authority, Merseyside. Senior House Officer to Dr Moss at Exminster Hospital in November 1986, and thereafter at EMC until February 1987.

Dr J. Eadie, SHO to Dr Conway, Moorhaven Hospital.

Dr Huw Edwards, consultant psychiatrist, Glangwili, Carmarthen, South Wales, 1978.

Dr Derrick Ellis, retired consultant psychiatrist. Medical member of MHRTs in September 1986 hearing application for the absolute discharge of Andrew Robinson, on 15 December 1986 after his readmission to Exminster Hospital, and on 17 October 1989 when application for discharge of Guardianship Order refused.

Dr Tim Exworthy, senior registrar in forensic psychiatry, Broadmoor Hospital, 1993, author of the model Assessment Report on Andrew Robinson (see Appendix 2).

Dr Patrick Gallwey, psychoanalyst and consultant forensic psychiatrist, in private practice since 1993. RMO to Andrew Robinson at the Butler Clinic (Regional Secure Unit) from February to August 1989.

Dr Christopher Gillespie, consultant general psychiatrist, specialist in rehabilitation. RMO for patients in long-stay hospital/hostel, called in by Dr Moss to review Andrew Robinson's medication on 16 August 1989.

Dr John Hambly, SHO to Dr Conway in 1986.

Dr Graham Lockerbie, Andrew Robinson's GP in Dartmouth circa 1988, who declined to give evidence to the Inquiry.

Dr Stuart McLaren, consultant general psychiatrist, RMO for Andrew Robinson in the community from April 1993, then during his detention in the Edith Morgan Centre from June to September 1993.

Dr William Monteiro, consultant general psychiatrist at South Devon Healthcare Trust. RMO for Andrew Robinson in the community from January to March 1993.

Dr Roger Moss, consultant general psychiatrist, retired at the end of 1992. RMO for Andrew Robinson during admission to Exminster Hospital and the Edith Morgan Centre from November 1986 to May

1987, and thereafter in the community until December 1987. Became the RMO again during admission to Edith Morgan Centre from November 1988 to February 1989, and on discharge from the Butler Clinic to the Edith Morgan Centre in August 1989. Andrew Robinson's consultant in the community (including during guardianship order) from November 1989 to December 1992.

Dr Richard Orr, consultant general psychiatrist. RMO for Andrew Robinson during admissions to the Edith Morgan Centre in December 1987, and May-June 1988.

Dr Roger Parke, senior registrar in psychiatry, EMC, 1988.

Dr Nancy Pears (deceased), consultant psychiatrist, Exe Vale Hospital. Andrew Robinson's RMO from July 1981, when he was transferred there from Broadmoor Hospital, until February 1983.

Dr Mark Selman, SHO to Dr Monteiro, September 1993. Gave first aid to Georgina Robinson immediately after the assault.

Dr John Speake, Andrew Robinson's GP in Torquay, who declined to give evidence to the Inquiry.

Dr B.G. Steggles, Tavistock GP.

Dr David Tidmarsh, consultant forensic psychiatrist at Broadmoor Hospital. Examined Andrew Robinson at HM Prison Cardiff in August 1978, and made psychiatric report on 31 August 1978. Recommended Andrew Robinson's committal to Broadmoor under section 60/65 Mental Health Act 1959.

Dr Edgar Udwin, retired consultant forensic psychiatrist. RMO for Andrew Robinson in Broadmoor Hospital from 1978 to 1981.

Dr Joseph Vella, psychiatric trainee, duty junior doctor at Edith Morgan Centre on 31 August 1993. Last doctor to see Andrew Robinson before incident on 1 September 1993.

Dr Jon Wride, General Practitioner. SHO at Edith Morgan Centre from August 1989 to February 1990. Community Medical Officer in psychiatry, based at Culverhay from August 1992 to December 1993.

Psychologists

Tony Black, retired consultant clinical psychologist, author of a psychological assessment on Andrew Robinson in October 1980.

Nick Caverner, principal clinical psychologist, assessed Andrew Robinson on 13 June 1986.

Community Nurses, South Devon

John Camus, enrolled mental nurse, South Devon Healthcare Trust. Nurse at Exminster Hospital in 1986, manager at Britannia Drop-In Centre, Paignton in 1987, and nurse with Paignton Community Rehabilitation Team from 1991. Andrew Robinson's community psychiatric nurse during his period under Guardianship, and involved in his care at EMC from June to September 1993.

Mike Gagg, community psychiatric nurse. Based at Waverley House, Torquay.

Les Grainger, community psychiatric nurse. Andrew Robinson's key worker under Guardianship Order, 1989-1992. Refused to give evidence to the Inquiry.

Iain Tulley, registered mental nurse, Community Services Manager, Plymouth and Torbay Health Authority. Senior nurse (Rehabilitation) at Cypress Hostel, 1987-1988. Knew Andrew Robinson in April 1987 when Andrew was referred for residential place at Cypress Hostel.

Jackie Wright (née Boyd), senior manager at Cypress Hostel. Working at Cypress as CPN from June 1987.

Social Workers, Devon Social Services

Steven Driscoll, social worker. Andrew Robinson's ASW from November 1985 to September 1986.

Peter Gleeson, principal social worker, Moorhaven Hospital, Andrew Robinson's social worker, April to November 1985.

Michael Hooper, principal social worker, Moorhaven Hospital, 1983-1985. Andrew Robinson's social worker in the community from March 1983 to April 1985.

Robert Steer, social worker at Culverhay from 1988 to 1992. Care manager of Guardianship Order from 1989 to 1992.

Landladies

June Hatsell, Andrew Robinson's landlady in Torquay from September 1992 to July 1993.

Carol Moore, Andrew Robinson's landlady in Paignton from June to November 1988, and from November 1989 to April 1990.

Others

Mrs. A., parishioner of the Rev. Peter Robinson, 1986-1989.

Anthony Dark, retired police inspector, Devon and Cornwall Constabulary. Inspector at Dartmouth Police Station in late 1988.

Miss B., victim of assault by Andrew Robinson in 1978 at Lampeter University, leading to the imposition of a restriction order and his detention in Broadmoor.

Thomas Dennis, lay member of the Mental Health Review Tribunal, 19 September 1986

Mr and Mrs Hopkins, managers of PIP Printing, Torquay, during 1993.

John Hansell, Dartmouth solicitor. Acted for Mrs A. from 1988 to 1989.

Marian Ingram, friend of Mrs Jennifer Robinson, who made regular visits to Andrew Robinson at his mother's request during his stay at his parents' home in Sidmouth in late 1992 and early 1993.

Neil Lindup, Day Services Development Worker, MIND in East Devon, Ottery St Mary, 1992-1993.

John Maundrell, friend of Andrew Robinson at Lampeter University at the time of the assault upon Miss B. in 1978. Made a statement to the police about the assault.

Judge Henry Palmer, circuit judge, president of MHRT for Andrew Robinson on 19 September 1986 and 17 October 1989.

Michael Pethick, friend of Andrew Robinson and resident in adjoining flat in 1992-1993.

Lady Rashleigh, family friend of Andrew Robinson, who took an active interest in his condition and treatment during his period of conditional discharge, 1982-1985.

Tony Unsworth, friend of Andrew Robinson at Lampeter University at the time of the assault upon Miss B. in 1978. Made a statement to the police about the assault.

Phillip Wilson, electrical department supervisor, Plymouth and South Devon Cooperative Society, Torquay. Sold the Prestige kitchen knife on 25 August 1993 to Andrew Robinson, the weapon used on Georgina Robinson on 1 September 1993.

South Devon Healthcare Trust – Management

Tony Boyce OBE, Chairman of South Devon Healthcare Trust.

Dr Margaret Cork, appointed Director of Mental Health, 1 August 1994.

Hilary Cunliffe, Director of Nursing and Patient Services. Commissioned an internal inquiry into the death of Stephen Hext.

Robin Foster, Assistant Director (Patient Services). Member of internal inquiry into the death of Stephen Hext.

Carole Heatly, Business Manager, Mental Health Directorate. Member of internal inquiry into the death of Stephen Hext.

Dr Ian McLeod, consultant in child psychiatry. Clinical Director of Mental Health, South Devon Healthcare Trust, February 1993 to July 1994. Member of internal inquiry into the death of Stephen Hext.

Dr John Lambourn, consultant psychiatrist. Medical Director, Mental Health Directorate since 1 August 1994.

Anthony Parr, Chief Executive, South Devon Healthcare Trust.

Pam Smith, temporary Director of Mental Health, April 1994-August 1994.

William Warr, Nurse advisor, mental health and operational service manager, Edith Morgan Centre.

Glossary and Abbreviations

ASW	Approved Social Worker
CMHT	Community Mental Health Team
CPA	Care Programme Approach
CPN	Community Psychiatric Nurse
DGH	District General Hospital
DH	Department of Health
ECA	Extra Care Area
EMC (or EMU)	Edith Morgan Centre (Edith Morgan Unit)
FHSA	Family Health Service Authority
GMC	General Medical Council
GO	Guardianship Order
HO	Hospital Order
MHA	Mental Health Act
MHAC	Mental Health Act Commission
MHRT	Mental Health Review Tribunal
MIND	National Association for Mental Health
NHS	National Health Service
NHSE	National Health Service Executive
NSF	National Schizophrenia Fellowship
OT	Occupational Therapy(ist)
RMO	Responsible Medical Officer
RSU	Regional Secure Unit
SDHT	South Devon Healthcare Trust
SHO	Senior House Officer
SHSA	Special Hospitals Service Authority
SSD	Social Services Department
UKCC	United Kingdom Central Council for Nursing, Midwifery and Health Visiting

Establishments

Broadmoor	Special Hospital
Butler Clinic	Regional Secure Unit
Cypress	Cypress Hostel, owned by SDHT
Culverhay	Community Mental Health Centre, Paignton
St Andrew's Lodge	Privately run hostel in Paignton
Waverley	Community Mental Health Centre, Torquay

Chronology of Andrew Robinson's Mental Health

EARLY LIFE 1957 – 1978

Nov. 28
1957
Andrew Robinson was born in Natal, South Africa, where his father had a parish. He attended two primary schools in Natal. The family spent a year in England and Andrew attended a day school in Herefordshire. When he was 9 the family returned to South Africa, and he attended a boarding prep school in Pietermaritzburg. When he was 12, the family returned to the UK and he attended West Buckland School, a Devon boarding school. He obtained 9 'O' levels and 3 'A' levels.

1976
In October Andrew Robinson attended Lancaster University, studying economics. Became preoccupied with his nose and in the winter vacation referred himself to a plastic surgeon in London who operated on his nose. He did not return to Lancaster University. In the summer of 1977 he worked in a camp site in France.

1977
In October Andrew Robinson went to St David's Lampeter to read French. After 2 weeks there he met Miss B., a fourth-year student with whom he had a brief relationship.

INDEX OFFENCE: FIRST HOSPITAL-RESTRICTION ORDER

1978

June 3
The index offence.

21
Dr Huw Edwards (Psychiatric Unit, West Wales Hospital) concluded that Andrew Robinson was suffering from a personality disorder and was definitely not psychotic.

Aug. 29
Andrew Robinson examined in HMP Cardiff by Dr Tidmarsh from Broadmoor Hospital, who diagnosed schizophrenia.

Sept. 26
Hospital Order with Restriction Order under MHA 1959 imposed following conviction for carrying a firearm with criminal intent and assault occasioning actual bodily harm. Admitted to Broadmoor Hospital.

TRANSFER TO LOCAL HOSPITAL FROM BROADMOOR

1981

July 15   Transferred to Exe Vale/Wonford Hospital, Exeter, under care of Dr Pears.

1982

Apr. 19   Went to live with his parents at Marystowe Vicarage, Lifton, near Tavistock.

Nov. 11   First seen by Dr Conway at Tavistock Hospital, referred from Exe Vale Hospital.

Dec. 2   Report from Dr Pears to the Home Office, saying that there was no evidence of active psychosis, and that Andrew Robinson had remained well.

CONDITIONAL DISCHARGE 1983-1986

1983

Jan. 27   Conditionally discharged from Restriction Order by the Home Office.

Feb. 24   Dr Conway became RMO.

May 27   Andrew Robinson's son born.

June 26   Case reviewed by Dr Conway. Noted to be managing very well, and contemplating move to Plymouth.

July 1   Report from Mike Hooper to Home Office, expressing concern about Andrew Robinson's attitude to women.

Aug. 25   Miss B. wrote to Broadmoor expressing concern that Andrew Robinson had been released.

1984

Aug. 18   Lady Rashleigh, a family friend in Devon, wrote to Dr Conway expressing concern about Andrew Robinson's preoccupation with his nose.

Oct. 31   Andrew Robinson's father wrote to Dr Conway asking if anything could be done about the side-effects of the drugs.

Dec. 3   Dr Conway saw Andrew Robinson and his parents, and 'was entreated to take the patient off all medication as it was felt that it was affecting him adversely ...'.

1985

Jan. 4   Seen by Mike Hooper, social worker. Andrew was noted to be very depressed.

10   Letter from Dr Steggles, GP, to Dr Conway saying that Andrew Robinson had become obsessed with his nose again, and was asking for Valium.

17   Noted by Mike Hooper to have improved after depot injection.

Mar. 14   Seen by Dr Conway, and said to be well. Noted to have been to
          Harley Street about further surgery to nose.

28   Andrew Robinson's father wrote to Dr Conway describing his
          son fidgeting after the injections. Andrew noted as being on
          Depixol 20 mg 4/52, and Dr Conway noted akathisia.

Apr. 24   Report by Mike Hooper, social worker, to Dr Conway following
          assessment of Andrew Robinson. He reported Andrew Robinson
          felt better since stopping his medication, and they had estab-
          lished a rapport.

Aug. 6   Letter from Rev. Robinson to Dr Conway, reporting Andrew
          Robinson as aggressive, deteriorating, and self-obsessed.

8   Seen by Dr Conway. Noted as well. Living at Lady Rashleigh's
          house.

Oct. 11   Seen by Dr Conway, and noted to be on no medication.

Nov. 12   Letter from Andrew Robinson's father to Dr Conway, expressing
          continued fears about his son's mental health, the suitability of
          bed-sit accommodation, and asking for sheltered housing.

1986
Jan. 27   Letter from Andrew Robinson's landlady at Greenbank Avenue,
          St Jude's, Plymouth (bed and breakfast accommodation) to Dr
          Conway, in which she described an incident in which Andrew
          Robinson rushed downstairs and handed them a knife and a
          tape of a conversation with Lady Rashleigh.

Mar. 10   Letter from Steve Driscoll to the Home Office, following inter-
          view with Andrew Robinson. He reported bizarre behaviour, and
          that he was concerned about Andrew Robinson.

Apr. 1   Letter from Andrew Robinson's father to Dr Conway, saying
          that Andrew Robinson was 'very ill, and should be receiving
          medication – possibly in hospital'.

ADMISSION TO MOORHAVEN HOSPITAL

Apr. 25   Admitted to Moorhaven Hospital, Plymouth, South Devon
          (RMO Dr Conway) under Section 3 of the MHA.

30   Report by Steve Driscoll to the Home Office, in preparation for
          the MHRT expressing his continued concern for Andrew Robin-
          son.

June 10   Dr Conway's first report to the MHRT.

Sept. 15 Dr Conway's second report to the MHRT. He reconfirmed his
          view that Andrew Robinson was not a paranoid schizophrenic,
          and that his behaviour had not been influenced or controlled by

> medication. Seen, but not examined psychiatrically, by Dr Ellis, medical member of MHRT.

16   Reported to be pestering nursing staff and coming 'close to striking' one of them (SP).

17   Section 3 rescinded by RMO. Andrew Robinson had already withdrawn his application to the MHRT.

19   Restriction Order discharged by MHRT (Judge Palmer, Dr Ellis, Mr Dennis). Andrew Robinson attended the hearing.

25   Andrew Robinson discharged from Moorhaven. Went to live with parents at Stoke Fleming near Dartmouth. Lived there for 2 months.

Oct. 24   Andrew Robinson's father wrote to Steve Driscoll, reporting that Andrew Robinson had smashed the radio into pieces, and shouted at his mother for listening to BBC Radio 4 as it was 'a neo-Nazi terrorist organisation'. He then attacked his father.

READMISSION TO AND DISCHARGE TO EXMINSTER HOSPITAL: FIRST ADMISSION TO EMC, NOVEMBER 1986

Nov. 18   Andrew Robinson was admitted to Exminster Hospital as an informal patient, under care of Dr Moss.

20   Took own discharge to a bedsit at 28 Pennsylvania Road, Exeter, against advice, Seen by Dr Moss, who did not feel that he could be detained under a section at that time.

21   Andrew Robinson arrested by Heavitree police after incident with mother, when he became angry with her for refusing to give him his passport so that he could leave the country.

22   Andrew's father wrote to Dr Moss protesting at the variance between the reports and Andrew's symptoms, and citing Andrew's obsession with radiation from Devonport Dockyard.

24   Andrew Robinson arrested by police in a restaurant, for eating a meal without the means to pay. Charged with obtaining property by deception, but matter not proceeded with.

28   Andrew Robinson thrown out of post office by Mr A., and on leaving made threats to harm Mrs A.

29   Admitted to EMC under Section 4, accompanied by police. He had gone to parents' home where he became violent; police were called to restrain him.

Dec. 1   Section 4 converted to Section 2 (RMO Dr Moss).

23   Section 3 order made (RMO Dr Moss).

1987

Apr. 22   Andrew Robinson admitted to Cypress Hostel on leave of absence from EMC.

May 22   Expiry of Section 3. Andrew Robinson leaves Cypress and goes to 24 St John's Road, Exeter.

SECOND ADMISSION TO EMC

Dec. 18   Andrew Robinson admitted to EMC under Section 2. Placed in Extra Care Area (RMO Dr Orr).

23   Transferred to open ward from ECA.

27   Absconded from EMC.

31   Returned to EMC by Exeter police.

1988

Jan. 5   Andrew Robinson restarted depot medication, after he had refused clopixol.

18   Section 2 expired. Andrew not felt to be suitable for further detention (Dr Orr). Discharged to a bed and breakfast in Paignton.

May 3   Father wrote to Dr Orr, saying that Andrew was again very paranoid.

THIRD ADMISSION TO EMC

May 9   Andrew Robinson informally admitted to EMC – not taking medication, under care of Dr Moss.

June 24   Formally discharged from EMC, after taking own discharge. Returned to bedsit in Paignton.

July 20   Seen by Dr Moss at Culverhay.

Aug. 2   Seen by Jackie Boyd, CPN. Andrew refusing to take medication or make any formal contact with community team.

Oct. 20   Andrew Robinson's landlady (Carol Moore) found a gun in his room. Iain Tulley gave air pistol and one cartridge to police.

Nov. 3   Father wrote to Dr Moss, reporting that Andrew was again very unwell, and that after 5 months without medication he was starting to hallucinate.

10   Arrested by Torquay police for making threatening telephone calls and sending letters to Mrs A. Seen by Dr Moss at police station – recommended admission under Section 2.

FOURTH ADMISSION TO EMC

Nov. 11   Admitted to EMC under Section 2 (RMO Dr Moss). Not taking any medication on admission.

25   First letter from John Hansell, Mrs A.'s solicitor, regarding her concerns about Andrew Robinson.

Dec. 8   Detained on Section 3, Dr Moss noting 'with a view to guardianship'.

9   Mrs A.'s solicitor, John Hansell, wrote to Dr Moss, indicating extreme concern for her safety, and seeking a meeting with Dr Moss.

13   Dr Moss noted 'We have now seen a letter he has written to Mrs A., almost certainly since admission. It indicates thought pattern far more sinister than he is revealing on the surface ...'.

20   Dartmouth police (Insp. Dark) wrote to EMC again seeking to be informed if Andrew Robinson released. Noted that Andrew Robinson now had Mrs A.'s address.

1989
Jan. 4   Letter from Dr Lockerbie (Andrew Robinson's GP) to Dr Moss, recording obsession with Mrs A.

6   Letter from Dr Moss wrote to John Hansell, indicating that there was no intention to release Andrew Robinson at this stage.

10   Letter from Insp. Dark to Dr Moss, setting out the full story of Andrew Robinson's dealings with Mrs A., and his bizarre behaviour in the village.

Feb. 1   Dr Moss wrote to Dr Donovan of Butler Clinic, requesting an assessment of Andrew Robinson with a view to transfer.

10   Assessed by Dr Gallwey, forensic psychiatrist, Butler Clinic, who agreed admission to Butler Clinic.

TRANSFER TO BUTLER CLINIC

Feb. 13   Transfer to the Butler Clinic RSU, Dawlish, Devon RSU.

May 11   Seen by Dr Moss for review of Section 3.

June 6   Section 3 renewed.

15   Parole trip to Dawlish. Behaved appropriately towards female staff and members of the public.

July 20   Case conference, Butler Clinic. Dr Moss in attendance.

TRANSFER TO EMC (FIFTH ADMISSION)

Aug. 1   Transfer to EMC from Butler Clinic

3   Appeal lodged against Section 3

4   Seen by Dr Moss. Guardianship Order being considered.

Oct. 17   MHRT (Section 3): application refused. Case conference discussing Guardianship Order, with Les Grainger (CPN) and Rob Steer (social worker) as keyworkers.

DISCHARGE FROM EMC UNDER GUARDIANSHIP ORDER

Nov. 16   Discharged from EMC under Guardianship Order to a landlady (Carol Moore) in Paignton (43 Colley End Road), to attend Britannia Day Centre.

24   Andrew Robinson's father wrote to Mr Padfield at Social Services saying: 'We are pleased that a Guardianship Order has been placed on Andrew, and trust that it will be renewed as long as necessary ...'.

1990
Mar. 23   Rob Steer saw Andrew at Culverhay, and reported that he was complying with medication but little else, and remained a risk.

27   Evaluation by Les Grainger, who had been seeing Andrew weekly for 4 weeks.

Apr. 9   Major overdose of orphenadrine (70 x 5mg tablets). Admitted to intensive care unit at Torbay Hospital.

SIXTH ADMISSION TO EMC

Apr. 12   Transfer to ECA at EMC on request from intensive care unit because of difficulties in management. In acute confusional state.

DISCHARGE TO HOSTEL IN PAIGNTON

June 29   Discharge to St Andrew's Lodge, a privately run hostel in Paignton – maintained on depot anti-psychotic medication. Attending day centre.

Dec. 7   Guardianship renewed.

1991
Apr. 22   Andrew Robinson's application to MHRT, heard in his absence, to be discharged from Guardianship, refused.

MOVE TO A GROUP HOME

Aug.   Moved to a group home at Shirburn Road. Noted to be making progress. Clopixol 300 mg every 2 weeks 'without undue side effects'.

Nov. 26   Seen by Dr Moss. Improved, and generally cooperative.

1992
Jan. 28   Seen by Dr Moss. Improvement sustained.

June 9   Dr Moss wrote to David Padfield, Assistant Director Social Services, saying he was 'impressed with the slow but steady recovery ...'. Recommended removal of Guardianship Order and halving of medication.

July 17   Andrew asked to leave Shirburn Road because his cleaning and hygiene levels were unacceptable.

21   Plan supported by Rob Steer in letter to David Padfield: 'I believe that Andrew will continue to comply with the wishes of the community mental health team, and has indicated that he is happy to continue taking his medication ...'.

MOVE TO OWN FLAT IN TORQUAY

Sept. 7   Moved to Flat 2, Little Princes, Meadfoot Road, Torquay, owned by the Hatsells. Medication had been halved.

22   Seen by Dr Moss: '... agreed to reduce his Clopixol to 3 weekly'.

23   Dosage had been cut to 150 mg/2 weeks. Dr Moss noted need to monitor him closely.

Oct. 22   John Camus attended to give depot injection. Andrew refused full depot, and was given an injection of 75 mg instead of 150 mg.

Nov.   Parents away in South Africa. Andrew Robinson staying in their house.

12   Continuing to decline full dose of depot medication.

Dec. 9   Reduced dose of depot medication given.
1993
Jan. 4   Visit by John Camus to parents' house. Depot medication refused.

25   Seen by Dr Wride: 'Andrew is staying in Sidmouth until the beginning of March, he has been off all medication at his own request for 6/52'.

Feb. 14   Andrew Robinson was reported to the police after an incident when he followed an 11-year-old boy in Sidmouth.

ANDREW ROBINSON RETURNED TO FLAT IN TORQUAY

Feb. 15   John Camus wrote: 'Visited Andrew at home today, he was angry at having been stopped by the police and says he will not go back to Sidmouth ever again'.

18   Dr Wride saw Andrew Robinson at his flat, accompanied by John Camus.

Mar. 4   Parents return prematurely from South Africa.

8   Father wrote to John Camus: 'I am sure you are aware that, since ceasing to take medication last November, Andrew has become very unwell'.

9   Dr Monteiro and John Camus attempt to visit Andrew at home but not in.

12   Seen by Dr Monteiro at team base. John Camus wrote: 'Andrew was seen by our consultant today. Although psychotic, he was not as sick as we were led to believe'.

16   Transferred to Torquay Community Mental Health Team. Dr McLaren takes over care. Mike Gagg (CPN) to be keyworker.

30   Mr and Mrs Hatsell accepted control over Andrew's money at his request.

May 14   Andrew Robinson's mother wrote to Andrew Williamson, Director of Social Services, expressing serious concern about Andrew's mental state: 'He decided not to have any more depot injections in November and has steadily deteriorated'.

SEVENTH ADMISSION TO EMC

June 9   Readmitted under Section 4 to ECA at EMC, converted to Section 3 on 10 June (RMO Dr McLaren).

11   Seen by Dr McLaren, who recorded: 'No clear indications of dangerous, delusional material from what he is saying ... No special scrutiny indicated as yet'.

14   Commenced on long-acting depot injections after 3-day assessment period. Transferred from ECA to main unit.

24   Seen by Dr McLaren, who recorded: 'Remains prominently deluded, with strong persecutory element. No focus on staff/patients'.

29   Seen by Dr McLaren, who 'feels that medication is gradually working'.

July 6   Noted to be 'spending lots of money on printing an article with bizarre content'. Wandering in and out of unit without staff knowing where he was going, and telephoning Pip Printers repeatedly. Pip Printers asked Andrew Robinson not to telephone again. Transferred back to ECA.

July 8   Medication increased – chlorpromazine 200 mg.

13   Pip Printers asked to return all of Andrew Robinson's scripts to EMC.

14   Andrew Robinson requested 'time out' in ECA. Left 2 hours later.

Aug. 10   Oral medication stopped. Depot medication continued as before.

25   Andrew Robinson bought a knife from the Torquay Co-op. No nursing note of his leaving the unit.

27   Asked nursing staff for weekend leave away from EMC. Told he could go to Exeter for the day on Saturday, 28 August, but that he had to return by 8 pm.

28   Absconded from hospital without leave. Went to London.

30   His room at EMC searched by John Camus, to find any clue as to where he had gone. Suicide note found, addressed to John Camus. Kitchen knife not uncovered.

31   Andrew Robinson returned to EMC at around 4 pm.
           Seen by Dr Vella at 7 pm.

Sept. 1   2.30 – 3.00 pm conversation with John Camus. Appeared 'calm' and 'very settled after his trip to London'. Just before 4 pm Andrew Robinson telephoned his father, asking him to find the manuscript of his autobiography.

           4 pm attacked and fatally wounded Georgina Robinson at EMC.

Oct. 22   Committed for trial.

28   Admitted to Broadmoor on remand under Sections 48/49 of the MHA.

1994
Mar. 22   Andrew Robinson pleaded guilty to manslaughter of Georgina Robinson. Placed under a Hospital Order with Restriction Order (Sections 37/41), admitted to Broadmoor.

June 30   Inquiry team visit and interview Andrew Robinson (with his solicitor) at Broadmoor.

Part A

Introduction

I. Background to the Inquiry

I see no sin:
The wrong is mixed. In tragic life God wot,
No villain need be! Passions spin the plot:
We are betrayed by what is false within.*

The Chairman and his colleagues on the Board of the South Devon Healthcare Trust invited us to complement the review of mental health services, which we had completed earlier in the year, by conducting an Inquiry into the tragic incident at EMC on 1 September 1993. Both they and we contemplated an exercise whose ambit of inquiry would be suitably circumscribed (our terms of reference appear in Chapter II and Appendix 3).

Given the experience of the escalating costs of such public inquiries, none of us needed any incentive to keep the Inquiry within tolerable bounds. Our initial reaction was to draw a line as at 9 June 1993, when Andrew Robinson was compulsorily admitted, for the seventh and last time since November 1986, to EMC. We fondly imagined that it was entirely appropriate for us to confine our interest to the period of Andrew's care and treatment which covered the circumstances prevailing immediately before the fatal event of 1 September 1993. Such a cut-off point would, it seemed, amply complement our earlier review of the existing psychiatric inpatient facilities. It would allow us to look more closely at the physical environment of the Centre, to examine staffing levels, to assess the suitability of the regime and to gauge whether anything might have been done in the days and weeks of June, July and August 1993 to prevent the onset of tragedy.

Our initial response to the forthcoming task was first disturbed by what we heard during the final stages of the review hearings at Torbay in January 1994. It was expressed to us, especially by members of the voluntary organisations who kindly attended and participated in a meeting with a range of worried parents, former patients, voluntary workers and other interested parties, that Andrew Robinson's relatives and associates had, on numerous

* George Meredith, *Modern Love* (1862), xliii.

occasions during the early part of 1993, brought to the attention of the Community Psychiatric Services his deteriorating mental state. They said that for many months, at least following Andrew's parents' departure in November 1992 for three months' holiday in South Africa, there had been much anxiety about Andrew's condition and much frustration that mental health services had not, they felt, responded appropriately, to the point where Andrew's mental state had worsened considerably by the time of the admission to EMC in June 1993. They felt that if only the community services had responded more quickly and had intervened more swiftly, there might have been a chance of preventing the incident of 1 September 1993. Since Andrew's severely disturbed mental state – a regression to his previous psychotic condition of the 1980s – was a direct cause of his violent and fatal assault on Georgina Robinson, it seemed to us important (if not imperative) to establish how effectively Andrew had been cared for in the community in the months, or even years, preceding the final admission.

Our decision, at the time of delivering our report on the mental health services in March 1994 (and Andrew's conviction for manslaughter at Truro Crown Court on 22 March 1994), to extend the retrospective time scale of the foreshadowed public inquiry, was fortified by what began to be revealed, once the documentary evidence was uncovered and analysed. Because Andrew's admission to EMC in June 1993 was, in fact, his seventh admission since November 1986, it was obvious that the Centre's management of Andrew (including his care and treatment) over the last six to seven years had to be scrutinised. What was Andrew's condition during that time, and what arrangements were made for his care and treatment during the intervals when he was in the community and not hospitalised? As our report will indicate, the use of Guardianship from 1989-1992 (involving social and health workers employed by the Trust and its predecessor) was of particular interest to us in the light of current official and public requirements about registers of seriously mentally disordered persons and the prospect of legislation for supervised discharge orders.

The documentary material sent us scurrying back to 1986. Why, then, have we looked back even beyond 1986? When we examined more closely the documentation in the possession of the Trust (and its predecessors), under the able and astute eyes of our counsel, Oliver Thorold and Michelle Strange, it emerged that, from Andrew Robinson's time at Broadmoor in 1978 to Torbay in the 1980s and

1990s, the deficiencies in the mode and manner of communication – a factor starkly revealed in the circumstances leading up to the death of Jonathan Zito[1] – had produced its own crop of deficiencies. Nevertheless, while we have concentrated our Inquiry on the period following November 1986, we have cast our eyes back to the offence in June 1978 which led to Andrew Robinson's committal to Broadmoor (the index offence) in order to inform ourselves fully of his cycle of severe mental disorder, spanning nearly two decades, which culminated not only in the disaster to Georgina Robinson and her family, but also in the incessant distress of Andrew and his family. As one of us (EM) wrote in 1991: 'For parents, watching an adult child's disintegration with schizophrenia is often a more difficult tragedy to come to terms with than the death of a child in a traffic accident'.[2]

Indeed, we think it will often be appropriate in an inquiry into a homicide of this kind to consider the patient's history since mental disorder first manifested itself. A sound risk-assessment of a patient must involve a careful consideration of any previous conspicuous acts or indicators of dangerousness, and the precise circumstances in which they occurred. This plainly imposes a duty on successive clinicians to heed the patient's entire history. Where medication is an issue, the patient's previous response to drugs, or experience of their side-effects, must affect the strategy later.

In addition, not surprisingly, a patient's clinical course is affected by past treatment. A patient who has suffered long-term schizophrenia, with frequent relapses, will tend to have a poorer prognosis than one for whom consistent medication has maintained stability.[3] Each successive doctor will usually be provided with information from his or her predecessor, sometimes of good quality, sometimes not. The quality of information-transmission can crucially affect later decisions.

Thus, there will usually be a series of chapters in a patient's psychiatric history, with links of several kinds from one to the next. Later decisions are, or certainly should be, influenced by knowledge

[1] The Report of the Committee of Inquiry into the case of Christopher Clunis, chaired by Mrs Jean Ritchie, QC.
[2] Murphy, E., *After the Asylums: community care for people with mental illness.* Faber and Faber (1991), p. 107.
[3] Johnson, D.A.W., Pasterski, G., Ludlow, J.M., Street, K., Taylor, R.D.W., 'The discontinuance of maintenance neuroleptic therapy in chronic schizophrenia patients: drug and social consequences'. *Acta Psychiatrica Scandinavica* (1983), 67, pp. 339-52.

of what has occurred before. An inquiry limited by a cut-off date will be hampered in its twin essential tasks of eliciting the relevant facts and identifying the lessons to be learnt.

Given the scope of our Inquiry over the fifteen years 1978 to 1993, we have been enabled to derive some general conclusions about the nature and quality of mental health services available and administered to Andrew Robinson. In the process we have also been able to form judgments about mental health services for the severely mentally disordered and the conduct of the prime actors in the unfolding tragedy, the falling shadow.

The fatal incident of 1 September 1993 was inherently unpredictable. For reasons connected with the unlawful absence of Andrew Robinson from EMC on 25 August and 28-31 August 1993, the homicidal attack on Georgina Robinson with a knife was, in the circumstances described below, preventable. That there was a likelihood of some dangerous conduct by Andrew Robinson, as a consequence of the removal of the restriction order on 19 September 1986 by the Mental Health Review Tribunal, was foreseeable for all those who thereafter became responsible for his care and treatment. It was entirely predictable that one day Andrew Robinson, if he was not maintained on medication under proper supervision, would attack somone (probably a young woman) and that steps should and could have been taken to prevent such an eventuality. That the necessary steps were not taken is the burden of our report. Mrs Wendy Robinson (Georgina's mother) was not overstating the case when she told us that her daughter's life was sacrificed to the inadequate care and treatment provided by mental health policy and practice for the severely mentally disordered people in this country.

Throughout our Inquiry we have been acutely aware that the profound misery suffered by Georgina Robinson's family during those appalling five weeks in the autumn of 1993, and the death of Georgina which continues to blight their lives, has been matched by an enduring misery of a different kind suffered by the other Robinson family. Ever since Andrew Robinson was diagnosed as suffering from paranoid schizophrenia in 1978, the Rev. Peter and Jennifer Robinson have suffered the continuing, desperate worries of anxious parents. Their constant entreaties to doctors and social workers to respond to their experiences of their son's frequent mental breakdowns appeared to them to go unheeded. And now their, and Andrew's, future appears every bit as bleak as that of

Georgina's family. It was manifest to us that, within the confines of the Inquiry room in July 1994, the two families perceptibly shared a common grief, arrived at from different vantage points but combining a unified plea to mental health services for a better system of care and treatment. If their cries do no more than arouse policy-makers, managers of mental health services and professional carers to listen more attentively and appreciatively to those daily experiencing the manifestations of mental ill-health, the tragedy at EMC will not have been in vain.

During the hearings we were alerted to the Trust's swift response to our recommendation for the future of EMC, which had in its design and function contributed to the tragedy. We wrote to the Chairman on 1 August 1994:

> In our review into the mental health services of the South Devon Healthcare Trust, we concluded that the Edith Morgan Centre was inappropriate for having the kind of inpatient services which are required in the context of care and treatment taking place in the community, and where an increasingly small proportion of severely disturbed persons need to be provided with intensive care, asylum (in the best sense of that word) and security. To that end, it concluded that plans should be laid for the expansion of inpatient facilities away from the site of the District General Hospital, but recognised, however, that that could be only a long-term solution – perhaps 5 to 10 years ahead. We therefore stressed the need for a short-term solution, to remedy the seriously prejudicial effect on mental health care.
>
> Our proposal was the setting up of a working group under the direction of a project officer, to produce plans for a rapid, short-term modification of the Edith Morgan Centre. Two issues needed to be addressed: the health and safety of patients and staff; and the greater integration of staff teams, particularly with regard to the Extra Care Area. The Trust instantly took on board our proposal and appointed Mrs Pamela Smith as the project officer. It was not our business – nor did (or do) we possess the expertise to cost the necessary modification. That was a matter entirely within the function of the Trust.
>
> Without dilating upon the costings of different options for redesigning the Edith Morgan Centre, we are satisfied that, in terms of value for money, the Trust could provide a new purpose built inpatient facility on a part of the DGH site. We have been given a presentation by the architect of the design for the new building, and see no objection to the Trust proceeding with this alternative plan, so long as it, too, is seen as a short-term solution. Plans for reprovision of the current inpatient services, off the hospital site, should still go ahead. We are encouraged to find that a design for the new

building on-site has an eye to alternative uses, as and when the long-term solution is in place. The fact of ready adaptability of any new building to other purposes demonstrates the Trust's commitment to our proposal for community-based inpatient facilities by the end of the twentieth century, or thereabouts.

At the time of writing this report (30 November 1994), we see no reason to alter our view.

II. Conduct of the Inquiry

Sunlight is the best of disinfectants.*

We presented our report on the review of the mental health services of South Devon Healthcare Trust on 18 March 1994. The Trust published the report simultaneously with a press conference at Torbay on 19 April 1994, on which occasion we announced that we would be holding a preliminary hearing on 16 May 1994 to set out the procedure for the conduct of the Inquiry into the circumstances surrounding the death of Georgina Robinson. Our terms of reference for the Inquiry had been framed:

> To inquire into the circumstances leading up to and surrounding the admission of Andrew Robinson to the Edith Morgan Centre, Torbay, and the incident on the 1st September 1993 in which he fatally assaulted Georgina Robinson, who subsequently died on the 7th October 1993, and to consider the lessons and implications arising with a view to making suitable recommendations.

These were subsequently amended to include an inquiry into the case of Stephen Hext in so far as it touched on the question of leave of absence.

We have explained in Chapter I why we interpreted our terms of reference to include events stretching back to June 1978, when Andrew Robinson's psychiatric condition first attracted the attention of mental health services via the criminal process. Our traverse of the ups and downs of his mental ill-health has highlighted some important aspects of the mental health system and the management of mental health services which were informed by our review and have amplified what we described in it. In the event we are confident that there are some stark lessons to be learned for the future care and treatment of seriously mentally disordered patients, both in the community and in hospitals. We think that our report sufficiently identifies the weaknesses in the system and those aspects of management which we found to be deficient, and

---

* Justice Brandeis of the US Supreme Court (1856-1941) quoted in the *New York Times*, 15 February 1984.

we therefore consider it unnecessary either to apportion blame to any individual or to spell out what needs to be done in the form of specific recommendations. We hope that readers will fully appreciate a report that is critical of the system and the management of services, without having to censure anyone who provided care and treatment to Andrew Robinson as part of a multi-disciplinary and multiple service. And we trust that those individuals who underwent the perhaps unpleasant experience of giving evidence in the full glare of publicity will recognise that their efforts to prevent the tragedy of 1 September 1993 happening again helpfully exposed to us the various events. This was necessary so that we could perform our duty to probe the circumstances thoroughly and at the same time be fair to everyone – including the victims of the tragedy.

Trapped in a mental health system which by common consent is woefully short of perfection, both those administering the system and the professionals providing the patients' care and treatment are bound to function less effectively than the public rightly demands. In so far as we appear to criticise any individual, such criticism should, therefore, be viewed as the identification of errors of judgment, made in the context of the system's problems and limitations. What we have sought to do is to take the reader beyond any question of blame and to explain how and why deficiencies occur, and will continue to do so unless and until radical changes in the system and in the management of services take place.

Apart from two procedural matters (which are dealt with in Chapter III), we describe here the way in which we set about the Inquiry. We do so largely for the reason that there is currently a good deal of official discussion and public debate about the nature and style of public inquiries. Our experience is that each tragic event or social scandal that arouses in the public a lack of confidence in a particular area of public life dictates its own method of inquiry. We do not for a moment suggest that our Inquiry is a model. But there may be features of it that prove worthy of replication in a similar case for investigation.

In our acknowledgements to those who provided support to our Inquiry, we adumbrated the method we employed. We explain here that method and our reasons for adopting it. The preliminary hearing on 16 May 1994 was consistent with the practice of public inquiries of recent years. (We include the statement we made then, in Appendix 3 to this report.) It re-affirmed the overriding principle

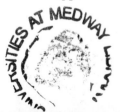

that a public inquiry is not like a piece of litigation between disputants. It is an investigation of what happened, why it happened and who was responsible for the happening. Lawyers have a distinct role to play in sifting the evidence, distilling and pinpointing the issues and promoting the interests of the inquiry body. They are not there primarily to promote the rights and interests of the parties they represent, although they will protect their clients consistently with their overall obligation to further the objectives of the inquiry.

The time-lag envisaged between the preliminary hearing and the hearing of oral evidence was eight weeks. Our experience was that even this period is barely adequate to ensure the collection of all the relevant documentation and the issue of letters to prospective witnesses. The problem in our case was that some delay was experienced while questions of confidentiality and disclosability of information were sorted out. Ordinarily, we think a period of 8-10 weeks from the date of the preliminary hearing should suffice. If necessary, the dates fixed for the public hearings should be postponed, but often this is not desirable. It is important to give the maximum amount of notice of the hearings. In doing so, some estimate of the time needed must be made. It is inconvenient, as well as costly, if the oral hearings run over the allotted time.

We announced the dates of our oral hearings for two four-day weeks at the end of July. In the event we sat to hear Mr Thorold's exegetic opening and the first three witnesses on 18 July 1994 and thereafter on 19, 20, 25, 26 and 27 July 1994. It had been our intention to sit on one more consecutive date to hear three witnesses from the management of the Trust. It had been found difficult for all three of them to be available on a single day at that time of the year. We therefore agreed to sit on one day – 22 September 1994 – to hear them. Their evidence came in two parts. The first was a detailed written statement compiled in response to questions which we had put to management. The postponement of their evidence from the end of July to the third week of September proved to be a bonus. It meant that a great many issues could be canvassed and disposed of without much, if any, oral questioning. We think that the splitting-off of evidence can be very fruitful in terms of reflective thought and shortened oral testimony. The second part was composed of amplified answers to questions not fully dealt with in the memorandum. Added to which, the management was able to furnish us with policy documents which had been

compiled after the events, one at least of them being in final draft
form only a few weeks before the oral hearings.

One novelty of the oral proceedings was the invitation to both
Robinson families to address us at the outset of the hearings, which
was gratefully accepted. Mrs Wendy Robinson, eloquently and with
commendable restraint, voiced her and her husband's feelings and
concerns about the failure of mental health services to prevent the
death of their daughter, Georgina. On the following morning (19
July 1994) the Rev. Peter Robinson spoke with similar, restrained
emotion, about the plight of his son Andrew. Unlike Mrs Wendy
Robinson, the Rev. Peter Robinson gave evidence by question-and-
answer. He was asked questions by Mr Thorold, Ms Davies and the
Chairman. We found both forms of giving evidence equally acceptable and helpful. Together their testimony to the tragedy to both
families set the tone of the Inquiry. The victims' need to assuage
the anguish of their bereavement or distress must be a paramount
consideration in any such inquiry. (Mrs Monica Hext, whose son
Stephen Hext died* on 15 December 1993 while absent from EMC
without leave, made a statement to us on 27 July 1994 at the
conclusion of the two-week session. We deal with the case of
Stephen Hext as part of Chapter XIV.) Mr and Mrs Hext also
attended the inquiry hearings throughout, maintaining a dignified,
attentive presence.

Since the central figure of the Inquiry was Andrew Robinson, it
seemed to us that we should interview him. We were conscious that
in the recent inquiry into the Beverley Allitt case, Sir Cecil Cloth-
ier, QC (a former Parliamentary Commissioner for Administration)
and his colleagues did not interview the nurse at Grantham Hospital who had killed and injured a number of children in her care
on the hospital ward. The Ritchie Inquiry team did, however,
interview Christopher Clunis and reported how helpful it was.
While in all three cases the individuals might prove unreliable
witnesses to their own misdeeds, owing to their mental disorder,
nevertheless we think that it is imperative that such a person
should be seen and heard. Accordingly, we three (together with our
counsel) visited Andrew Robinson at Broadmoor Hospital on 30
June 1994. He was assisted by his solicitor, Mr Richard Porritt,
who had persuaded his client to grant us the interview. An account
of the meeting, which lasted 1¾ hours, was read out to the oral
hearing on 19 July 1994. We indicated then that there were only

* The coroner's court returned an open verdict.

three items in the interview which we were disposed to take account of, without necessarily accepting the truth of what Andrew Robinson was saying. The first, and influential matter pertained to the apparent success of the Guardianship Order from 1989 to 1992. It was in the course of hearing about Andrew's attitude to his officially supervised medication during the currency of the Order that we learned of his communication with the Mental Health Act Commission. We later uncovered the correspondence which revealed Andrew's full understanding of his legal rights under the Order. (We deal with this significant element in the operation of a Guardianship Order in Chapter XII.) The second matter – of much less significance – was the reference to a letter about obtaining a firearms licence seen by a social worker when he visited Andrew in May 1993. The third matter provided confirmatory evidence of the lax practice about the unhindered movement of patients in and out of EMC, to which we allude in Chapter XIV.

We should mention briefly the one-day seminar which we held on 1 August 1994. The idea for identifying specific topics for general discussion and debate stemmed from the experience of two of us (LBC/EM) in the Ashworth Hospital Inquiry in 1991 (see Report of the Committee of Inquiry into complaints about Ashworth Hospital, Cm 2028-I, pp. 4-5). The papers delivered in the seminar were of such high quality that the publishers of this report have agreed to publish them separately in book form.

Hearings in public

We determined at the outset to conduct our proceedings in a public forum because we believe in the principle of openness whenever the public interest demands it. There was no objection to that; indeed we were encouraged by the Chairman of the Trust (presumably with the support of his fellow Trust Board members) to be as open-minded and open-handed about publicity as circumstances permitted. We guessed that the two Robinson families were highly desirous of a public proceeding, even if it meant a painful experience for them. In the result we gauged, accurately, that they greatly appreciated the opportunity not only to voice their own concerns, but also to hear the various witnesses give their evidence, sometimes under close questioning. Even though there is a transcript of the witnesses' evidence, which could be made available to any interested party (perhaps at some cost) it is never the same to read what was said, as it is to hear it from the mouths of the individual witnesses. Demeanour and manner in answering questions are important elements in testing the credibility of a witness's evidence.

The only hesitation in the general acceptance of openness in the Inquiry was the scope of media coverage. Following the traditional stance of the legal system, the journalist can come in and write unhindered. But modern technology, in the form of audio and video transmission and/or recording, somehow must not be allowed to function. Why is this?

Proceedings in courts in England and Wales – Scotland, unhampered by any legal provision, has recently sanctioned the televising of court proceedings – cannot be recorded and relayed either on radio or television; this is because the law prohibits any recording instrument being used in the courtroom. The law restricts the activity of the journalist to his pen and notepad. Section 41 of the Criminal Justice Act 1925 makes it an offence to take a photograph in court. This is not the only legal impediment to televising courtroom proceedings. Apart from that statutory provision, the taking of photographs or televising of proceedings would in some circumstances be a contempt. Courts also assert a general power, not very precisely defined, to control the proceedings. In exercise of this power a court could refuse to permit recording equipment to be present during hearings. It is the all-embracing nature of the statutory provision, however, that makes it the crucial obstacle to television coverage of the courtroom scene.

The history of the ban on photography in court is uncertain and obscure. But in recent times it has been both stoutly maintained by judges and administrators, and assailed by legal reformers. While there have been some incursions, in more or less limited forms, in the courts of North America, the courts in England have not yet succumbed to even experimental televising of court cases. Courts in other Anglo-Saxon legal systems have followed suit. Likewise, other quasi-judicial proceedings have been conducted in accordance with the practice of the courts of law. We are not aware that any Commission of Inquiry in the UK has been subjected to radio or television coverage, with the sole exception of Scotland. The most that has been allowed has been video-circuit television to accommodate an overflow of numbers of the public present at the Inquiry hearings. Indeed, Lord Justice Scott in his inquiry into the Iran arms deals specifically denied access to radio and TV to the public hearings.

Our approach to this problem has been dictated by the potential benefits that we see in it for the legal process and public understanding of it. The Royal Commission on the Press (the Ross Commission of 1949) wrote:

> The democratic form of society demands of its members an active and intelligent participation in the affairs of their community ... More and more it demands also an alert and informed participation not only in purely political processes but also in the efforts of the community to adjust its social and economic life to increasingly complex circumstances. Democratic society, therefore, needs a clear and truthful account of events, of their background and their causes. (Cd. 7700, para 362)

Radio and television provide the greatest potential for achieving just that 'clear and truthful account'. Why then not accept their powerful influences? A Chicago trial lawyer, who reluctantly succumbed to the experiment of television in the courtroom, expressed the opinion that as a result of television recording, the judges behaved better, the lawyers prepared and presented their cases more effectively and economically, and the public was incomparably better informed.

We therefore made it known that the tape-recorder and the television camera could be present throughout the public inquiry in Newton Abbot, so long as there was no physical obstruction to the orderliness of the proceedings. For what it is worth we record our impression of the effect of uninhibited media coverage at the Inquiry.

We are convinced of the public and professional benefit of permitting the broadcast of tribunal hearings. Any fears of physical obstruction were entirely misplaced: one single television camera, trained for the most part on the witness, soon went entirely unnoticed. No lights or other studio impediments were required. The witnesses were in no way flustered or deterred, or for the most part even conscious of the recording. We are confident that they remained untroubled that their evidence was going to be relayed to the populace. If they were aware, they raised no objections and showed no sign of disquiet, let alone dissent. There was a minor protest by the management witnesses on 22 September 1994; this was resolved by the voluntary withdrawal of the cameraman. We have experienced for ourselves the sense of Jeremy Bentham's argument in favour of open justice, namely that 'it keeps the judge, while trying, under trial'.

III. Evidence to the Inquiry

Testimonial exclusionary rules and privileges contravene the fundamental principle that 'the public ... has a right to every man's
evidence'.*

Only one person to whom we extended an invitation to give relevant
and important evidence declined to respond without advancing
some reason for so declining. Since the ability of non-statutory
inquiries to perform their task with the requisite thoroughness is
a perennial question that hovers over all public inquiries, we devote
a few words here to the disclosure of all relevant information for
the purposes of the Inquiry.

Mr Les Grainger, a community psychiatric nurse, was Andrew
Robinson's key worker, jointly with Mr Rob Steer, during the period
leading up to the discharge of the Guardianship Order in November
1989. Initially, we had difficulty in tracing Mr Grainger, but he was
tracked down, working in the Durham area. Contact with his
solicitor in Darlington revealed a distinct reluctance, and ultimately a refusal, on Mr Grainger's part to assist the Inquiry. This
was despite a full and detailed explanation to his solicitor of what
was expected of someone employed in a public service. Since, from
the helpful evidence of Mr Rob Steer and Mr John Camus, we were
able to cover the events adequately, we did not feel it was necessary
to pursue the role which Mr Grainger played in those events.

There was no legal compulsion upon Mr Grainger to assist us,
save for the strong professional obligation to further the public
interest in uncovering how and why a tragic incident occurred in
an inpatient psychiatric facility. It is entirely understandable that
workers in health and social care should feel reticent about giving
evidence to inquiries – particularly those which are conducted in
the full glare of the public. Over the years, social workers and
others in health care work have often been pilloried by the press
and discomforted publicly, and not always fairly, by criticism in
inquiry reports. Nevertheless, the hostility towards public inquiries cannot override the obligation to account for the service supplied

---

* *United States* v. *Bogen*, 339 US 323,331 (1950).

(or not supplied) to individuals. In many instances the sponsoring authority of the public inquiry will be the worker's employer, and can therefore order that worker to give evidence under the terms and conditions of that employment. (We are not aware that anyone in the employ of South Devon Healthcare Trust was in any way unwilling to come forward; on the contrary, it appeared to us that there was a keenness to help by way of, often very impressive, written statements and oral testimony.) But Mr Grainger was out of reach of any such direct compulsion. He could be persuaded to come forward only if he accepted it as his public duty.

Where a responsible sponsoring body – be it central or local government, or any other public institution – deems it necessary to order a public inquiry, anyone invited to give evidence should instinctively agree to help. For those who are professionally qualified, it cannot be doubted that it is their professional obligation to submit themselves to what is undeniably an uncomfortable experience. For the private citizen, there is no similar obligation. But if the public requires to know the truth about a public scandal, a natural disaster or some failure of a public service, the witness to some aspect of that event should likewise assist. Otherwise sponsoring authorities will have to plead for some statutory authority which will carry the power of sub-poena.

An altogether different kind of refusal to assist – because the refusal was reasoned – came from the medical profession. Two GPs – Dr John Speake from Torquay and Dr Graham Lockerbie from Dartmouth – were invited to give the Inquiry some important assistance. Dr Speake had been Andrew Robinson's GP during the first half of 1993 – until Andrew's admission. He was asked to provide medical records which would give some picture of Andrew's clinical condition before the fatal incident of 1 September 1993. Dr Lockerbie had appeared to be Andrew's GP following the discharge by the MHRT in September 1986 and Andrew's return to his parents' home at Stoke Fleming where he first developed his obsession with Mrs A., and later his delusional behaviour towards her.

At first Dr Lockerbie agreed to give oral evidence, but indicated his need to be supplied with copies of his notes which were held by Dr Speake. These notes were not at that time forthcoming without Andrew Robinson's consent to their release being first obtained. For reasons that we do not need to explain, Andrew, while having given his consent to the Inquiry to have a sight of hospital records over the years, declined to extend his waiver to confidentiality at the later stages of our pre-hearing preparations. On 17 June 1994 Dr Speake wrote to us as follows:

> Thank you for your letter dated the 6th June requesting medical information on my patient Mr Andrew Robinson. I have noted all your questions and I feel that most of them would be answered from his medical records. I am sure they will be most useful for your inquiry. I feel however, that I have a duty to protect my patient's confidentiality. I have no wish at all to be obstructive and I would be more than happy to release the records if I had either consent from the patient or an order from yourself compelling me to release them to the inquiry. I would welcome your help in this matter.

We explained to Dr Speake that as a non-statutory inquiry we had no power to compel him to attend to give evidence or to order him to produce any documents. But we sought to persuade him that principles of medical confidentiality did not inhibit him from (i) giving the Inquiry access to Andrew's GP records; (ii) giving evidence about any consultations with Andrew; or (iii) giving evidence about any information communicated to Dr Speake about Andrew. Our explanation for the view that confidentiality was overridden by the public interest in disclosure to the Inquiry did not persuade Dr Speake, and we proceeded without any medical notes from Dr Speake (which included GP notes dating back to at least 1986). Dr Speake wrote on 11 July 1994:

> Thank you for your letter of July 6th 1994. I have studied your comments in great detail. After careful consideration I feel it would be improper of me to provide you with a Medical Statement, appear at the inquiry or release Mr Andrew Robinson's notes. The main reason for this is because Mr Robinson himself declined to give consent ...
> I am sure you will be disappointed at my decision to decline giving medical information. From the General Practitioner's perspective I feel that confidentiality should be given the highest priority. I can assure you that I have given the matter my deepest consideration.

Our reasoning for the view that confidentiality did not demand non-disclosure to us ran along the following lines. The NHS Executive has issued Guidelines to Health Authorities and Trusts (NHS Executive HSG(94)27, 10 May 1994) which state under a heading 'If things go wrong':

33. If a violent incident occurs, it is important not only to respond to the immediate needs of the patient and others involved, but in serious cases also to learn lessons for the future ...

34. Additionally, after the completion of any legal proceedings it may be necessary to hold an independent inquiry. *In cases of homicide, it will always be necessary to hold an inquiry which is independent of the providers involved.*

36. In setting up an independent inquiry the following points should be taken into account:

    i. *the remit of the inquiry* should encompass at least:
      – the care the patient was receiving at the time of the incident;
      – the suitability of that care in view of the patient's history and assessed health and social care needs;
      – the extent to which that care corresponded with statutory obligations, relevant guidance from the Department of Health, and local operational policies;
      – the exercise of the care plan and its monitoring by the key worker.

There is in that official statement a clear public interest in the proper conduct of such inquiries. While the 'provider' can, of course, readily make available to the Inquiry those medical records which it holds, and which may convey much of the picture, it is inevitable that others (such as GPs) are likely to hold records or information to which access is necessary for the full picture to be understood. The inquiry process would be frustrated if principles of confidentiality prevented full access to records likely to be of relevance. Any inquiry into the clinical history of a homicidal patient with a diagnosis of schizophrenia, such as Andrew Robinson, must involve consideration of his clinical history and management over a period of years. Since in a case of long-standing schizophrenia, multiple relapses lead to poorer prognosis, the Inquiry will necessarily be concerned with the patient's entire clinical history. His GP records are likely to be the only available medical records for some periods of that history.

In the case of *W* v. *Egdell*[1] the Court of Appeal confirmed that there can be competing public interests, on the one hand, in the duty of confidentiality owed by a doctor to his patient, and on the other, in the disclosure of a report to third parties, and that the balance can favour the latter. In the course of the judgment the court referred to the GMC rules, citing an exception to the duty of confidentiality:

[1] [1990] Ch. 359.

81(g) Rarely, disclosure may be justified on the ground that it is in the public interest, which, in certain circumstances such as, for example, investigation by the police of a grave or very serious crime, might override the doctor's duty to maintain his patient's confidentiality.

A police investigation is given simply as an example. A public inquiry into Georgina Robinson's death presents similarly compelling grounds for the public interest in disclosure to predominate. At the end of the Court's judgment, Lord Justice Bingham (as he then was) said:

> There is one consideration which in my judgment, as in that of the judge, weighs the balance of public interest decisively in favour of disclosure. It may be shortly put. Where a man has committed multiple killings under the disability of serious mental illness, decisions which may lead directly or indirectly to his release from hospital should not be made unless a responsible authority is properly able to make an informed judgment that the risk of repetition is so small as to be acceptable ...

This passage gives proper recognition to the extent of the public interest in preventing homicides by mentally disordered individuals. Just as the independent forensic psychiatrist in *Egdell's case* was entitled to submit his report to the Home Office, even though he was hired by the patient for the purpose of assisting his case before the MHRT, so a GP would not be breaching any confidentiality if he were invited to disclose his patient's records to a properly-constituted public inquiry.

We trust that our view correctly states the legal position, If so, no future public inquiry into a grave criminal event involving a seriously mentally disordered person will be hampered by the failure to uncover all the relevant medical information pertaining to the past care and treatment of the patient.

We considered the current attitude of the two relevant professional bodies – the General Medical Council (GMC) and the United Kingdom Central Council for Nursing, Midwifery and Health Visiting (UKCC).

The GMC in its disciplinary role has always regarded itself as a quasi-judicial body and, therefore, hesitant about giving advice to its members. If it were consulted by a doctor about the propriety of disclosing medical notes to a public inquiry, it would refer the practitioner to his or her medical defence organisation, for example, the Medical Defence Union or Medical Protection Society. If the GMC was ever called upon, in the course of disciplinary proceedings, to pronounce upon disclosure of medical notes to a public inquiry, it would doubtless have to take into account the public interest. We are in no doubt ourselves that guidance on the matter would be extremely helpful. Just as in the case of police investigation of a very serious crime, the GMC has indicated – in rule 81(g) – that the public interest 'might override the doctor's duty to maintain his patient's confidentiality', so the dictates of a public inquiry should, likewise, exceptionally override confidentiality. Rule 81(g) might usefully be so amended.

The UKCC takes altogether a more robust and public-spirited attitude, although its powers inhibit enforcement. Giving evidence to a public inquiry falls squarely within the UKCC Code of Professional Conduct, which provides that nursing members should always serve the interests of society and 'promote and safeguard the well-being and interests of patients/clients'. The UKCC's disciplinary powers extend only to removal from the register, or a caution, the latter being administered only when mitigating circumstances are present to avoid removal from the register. Failure to give evidence to a non-statutory public inquiry would not be considered sufficiently serious to warrant the drastic sanction of removal from the register. The lack of any power in the UKCC to impose a lesser sanction leaves a gap in the disciplinary regime. Failure to give evidence at a public inquiry would have to be dealt with, if at all, through the terms and conditions of the contract of employment.

Public inquiries, whether statutory or non-statutory, need to be assured of optimum disclosure of information from all the relevant sources. Professional bodies, naturally sensitive to the safeguarding of confidential information, should readily concede the overriding public interest in disclosure to public inquiries.

The point was exemplified, with judicial authority, in the course of the Inquiry into complaints about Ashworth Hospital. The Committee of Inquiry ordered the Special Hospitals Service Authority to produce for inspection (and selection of the relevant documents) the personal file of a nurse against whom complaints of sexual impropriety towards a mental patient had been made. The SHSA declined to disclose the file on the ground that there was a public interest immunity from disclosure in respect of a class of documents consisting of the files of nurses employed in Special Hospitals. Confidentiality in such files was claimed. On the judicial review of the Committee's order for disclosure, Mr Justice Schiemann established the principle that 'subject to national or public security, the inquiry body is entitled to demand production to itself of all relevant material and to decide for itself whether the whole, or part only, of the material should be publicly disclosed'.[2]

[2] *Report of the Committee of Inquiry into Complaints about Ashworth Hospital.* Cm. 2028 I & II (1992), ch. VI, p. 32 and Appendix 6J, pp. 339-44.

Part B

Events at the Edith Morgan Centre, August/September 1993

IV. The Fatal Event

Between the acting of a dreadful thing
And the first motion, all the interim is
Like a phantasma, or a hideous dream.*

At about four o'clock in the afternoon on 1 September 1993 a female patient at EMC was discussing her programme for the next two days with a member of staff, an occupational therapist, Miss Georgina Robinson, in a four-bedded dormitory on the first floor of the building. Through the open door of the dormitory there suddenly appeared, unattended and unobserved, a male patient, Mr Andrew Robinson (no relation), who occupied a bedroom on the same floor some distance away from the dormitory. The female patient, who alone witnessed the ensuing incident, described the unprovoked and frenetic attack on Miss Robinson by Mr Robinson first clutching her round the top half of her body below the neck and then inflicting on the unsuspecting, struggling and screaming victim multiple stab wounds, seven in all, with a kitchen knife to the back and side of her neck, face and shoulder blade. Miss Robinson suffered major trauma to her carotid artery and jugular vein. She was dragged off the bed where she had been sitting and was further stabbed while kneeling on the floor. The fact that she managed to survive for five weeks is a tribute to the efficacious first aid carried out by Dr Selman, a Senior House Officer, together with a community psychiatric nurse and another nurse. Having been agitatedly summoned by the female patient, they rushed to the scene. They resuscitated Georgina and stabilised her condition. She was taken for immediate surgery and thereafter into intensive care, unhappily to no avail. For most of the following five weeks she was conscious and must have undergone pain and suffering. On 7 October 1993 she died.

In her statement made on behalf of Georgina Robinson's family (to which we referred in Chapter II), Mrs Wendy Robinson told us that the family had admired and wondered at Georgina's determination to live 'despite the pain to overcome the paralysis her

---

* *Julius Caesar* II.1.63-5.

injuries had caused, to find ways of communicating as her vocal chords had been damaged. She had to cope with the memory and trauma of such an unprovoked, vicious and cruel attack during the five weeks, which', Mrs Robinson graphically stated, 'will be etched in our minds forever'.

Some five minutes before the fatal incident, Andrew Robinson had telephoned his father, according to whom he had engaged in a desultory conversation about a manuscript of his, entitled 'Victim of the Magic Circle', which had gone missing and could not be discovered at his parents' home. Whatever that short conversation may have evoked in Andrew – and nothing that we have heard would indicate any arousal, even in someone suffering from a psychotic illness – he went immediately to fetch the knife which (as we shall describe) he had purchased a few days earlier in Torquay. In a tape-recorded interview on the day following the incident Andrew stated: 'I felt the only way to escape my problem which involved psychiatry was a drastic course of action, it just happened. I wasn't angry or anything ....' He went on to refer, however, to the loss of the manuscript which he had compiled, saying: 'I went up to her. I thought I had to get out of the problem. I lost my manuscript, the vital manuscript, it was my whole life, my whole soul.' We conclude that the fact of the missing manuscript triggered off the effusion of his dangerous, psychotic behaviour. It cannot be inferred that, had the manuscript been to hand (or at least readily accessible) the ensuing behaviour would have been averted. There is nothing that suggests that the attack was in any way premeditated, specific-related or even gender-related, although his past antipathy towards women indicates that the victim would probably be female. So far as anyone can tell, neither assailant nor victim knew the other. Miss Robinson had been employed at EMC during the period of Andrew Robinson's detention, but she had had no clinical or other responsibility for his care and treatment. The attack was entirely random, motiveless and senseless. It was the manifestation of a patient's serious mental illness. Dr Joseph Vella, who was the junior doctor on duty the previous evening, and hence the last medically qualified person to see Andrew, described him as still suffering from the psychotic illness that prompted his compulsory admission in June 1993.

Andrew Robinson's absences from EMC were frequent and unauthorised. We describe the pattern of intermittent absenteeism relating to the ten days before the fatal event, including relevant individual contacts. On Sunday, 22 August he was visited at the Centre by his father. Mr John Camus, a psychiatric nurse who had since 1989 played a sustained and, spasmodically over the last nine months, very supportive role in Andrew's life, said that it was unusually 'a good meeting'. The next day Andrew rang his father asking for financial assistance to pay for an advertisement promoting a pamphlet along the lines of the missing manuscript. Back in June and July he had been in touch with a printer in Torquay seeking the type-setting of a short document. The printer had become perturbed at its content and sent it to the hospital authorities. He recalled that Andrew Robinson had visited the print shop on two or three occasions, invariably unescorted.

Likewise, Andrew Robinson's acquaintance, who occupied an adjoining flat in the house in Torquay whence Andrew had come into EMC, spoke of visits 'on most days'. Mr and Mrs Hatsell, the landlords at the address, spoke of Andrew 'popping in fairly regularly until Saturday, 28 August 1993 when he came asking for £60'. (Mrs Hatsell had, since March 1993, looked after Andrew's money, at the request of Andrew's mother. On that occasion she had given him £40.) The nursing note for 30 August confirms the visit two days before, adding that Andrew 'left without going down to his flat' in the basement of the house. That unescorted visit came during an absence from EMC which began on that day and ended with his unaided return on Tuesday, 31 August 1993. Andrew Robinson told us that he went into Torquay most days: 'Sometimes I'd get permission. Sometimes I just went. Other patients would do the same.'

Before the final bout of absenteeism, there had been a significant, unescorted visit by Andrew Robinson to the shopping centre in Torquay. On Wednesday, 25 August 1993 (for which day there is not even a record of his being away from the hospital), at around 4.30 pm, he made two separate purchases in the electrical department of the South Devon Co-operative Society. The first was a Teflon saucepan and two mugs. These items were found by John Camus in Andrew's bedroom when he 'searched' it on the evening of Monday, 30 August. The second was not uncovered during the search. This was a Prestige stainless-steel kitchen knife, which became the homicide weapon. It would be reasonable to infer that the knife was left at Andrew's flat, probably later that day, and that he recovered it some time during his absence from EMC during the period 28-31 August, and took it to EMC on his return there the night before the fateful day, that is, subsequent to John Camus's search of his room. Andrew Robinson stated in a letter to us that he had concealed the knife in a suitcase in his room at EMC. There is no evidence to corroborate Andrew's statement.

The nursing notes for this period show that on 27 August Andrew sought permission to 'go out for the day tomorrow – he has been told to be back by 8 pm'; Mr Camus's note for the following day recorded that he 'had not returned from visit at time of hand-over, 8.10 pm'. For 29 August 1993 the note states: 'not returned from agreed day leave'. An entry for 1 pm on 29 August states that the police were contacted 'to stress the importance of contacting Andrew's parents in Sidmouth, not only for any safety issues (given his past history) but also to inform them he is missing'.

In the absence of any hospital-prescribed procedure for the grant of leave of absence, the various excursions to Torquay and presumably elsewhere (London, in the case of the weekend of 28/29 August) were made either on the basis of a 'by-your-leave', or with express permission of, probably senior, nursing staff. Such visits outside EMC – unescorted, to boot – were clear breaches of Section 17 of the Mental Health Act 1983. We do not pause here to consider the persistent non-compliance with this statutory provision, save to say that it appears to us that the fatal assault on Georgina Robinson on 1 September 1993 by the means of the recently-acquired knife, purchased during an unauthorised absence, and thereafter brought to EMC, was a direct consequence of an unlawful act by those employed by South Devon Healthcare Trust.

Andrew Robinson was subsequently charged with the murder of Georgina Robinson at Truro Crown Court on 22 March 1994 before Mr Justice Drake and a jury. Initially he sought to set up a defence of justifiable homicide and this was summarily rejected by the judge. He altered his plea to guilty to manslaughter on the grounds of diminished responsibility. A Hospital Order was made with a restriction order unlimited in time, and he was admitted to Broadmoor Hospital, to which he had already been transferred from prison on 28 October 1993, and where he had been from 1978 to 1981 as a result of a serious event in 1976. We turn now to the beginning of the story.

Part C (1)

Andrew Robinson's Socio-psychiatric History, 1978-1986

V. The Index Offence

> The simple dichotomy of the law that an offender either is, or is not,
> responsible for his offences has produced grave moral and legal
> anomalies.*

By any standard of human conduct, the incident at St David's,
Lampeter on 3 June 1978 was extremely serious. It was a highly
dangerous – indeed, homicidal – attack with a loaded shotgun on
a young woman by a seriously mentally disordered young man,
subsequently diagnosed as suffering from paranoid schizophrenia.
On the basis that the best predictor of future behaviour is the
individual's past behaviour, this 'index offence' was of immense
significance to anyone who was subsequently to be called upon to
decide on Andrew Robinson's future care and treatment, as well as
to determine any discharge from restrictions on his liberty. On the
day of the shooting, Andrew Robinson had taken a shotgun from
the room of a fellow student, Tony Unsworth. Mr Unsworth went
looking for Andrew and found him hiding in the toilet, whereupon
Andrew ran off. Mr Unsworth searched for him, concerned for
Andrew's safety. His statement to the police gave a full account:

> I again looked for him in the new buildings ... Whilst there Andrew
> returned. He stood in the doorway holding a bottle by its neck in a
> threatening manner. I asked him to tell me where the gun was. He
> replied 'Don't do this, you're the last person I want to do this to'. On
> hearing this I assumed he was going to hit me with the bottle and I
> slammed the door in his face ... John Maundrell ... and I ran after him.
> We chased him ... When at a distance of about fifty yards from him I
> saw Andrew stoop down and pick up the shotgun from the undergrowth
> nearby. He then loaded the shotgun. I shouted at him to put it down.
> He took no heed, and as I assumed he might use the shotgun on me
> I started walking away from him. As I did so I heard the gun being
> fired and I turned around, as I knew it was only a single barrel. He
> again reloaded and came towards us. On seeing this I ran off and
> locked myself in one of the New Building rooms with John Maundrell.
> After a period of about fifteen to twenty minutes when leaving the
> room we were told that Andrew had been arrested ...

---

* Barbara Wootton, 'Crime and the Criminal Law', *Selected Writings*, vol. 2: *Crime
and the Penal System I*, Macmillan (1992), p. 57.

Andrew Robinson had gone to the room of Miss B. with the loaded shotgun. She was a fourth-year student with whom he had become infatuated and had a short-lived affair. The relationship was described by Dr Tidmarsh (Consultant Psychiatrist, Broadmoor) in his report of 31 August 1978 to the Crown Court, Swansea, where Mr Robinson was convicted on 7 September 1978 of carrying a firearm with intent:

> 2 weeks after his arrival in October 1977 he met and became infatuated with a fourth-year student, [Miss B.]. It seems that she suggested sexual intercourse but his premature ejaculation led her to terminate the relationship very soon afterwards. From then on his mind dwelt obsessively on her, at times he considered her perfect and at other times he hated her and wanted to disfigure her, blaming all his misfortunes on his nose ... On 21.11.77 while in a state of depression and agitation he took a substantial overdose of paracetamol and aspirin. He was admitted for 8 days to the psychiatric unit of the West Wales General Hospital. On discharge he returned home where he remained tense, depressed and obsessed with the desire to smash [Miss B.'s] face in with a brick, an act which he rehearsed in the garden.

Miss B.'s statement to the police recorded the incident as follows:

> I heard a shot coming from the side of the Arts building. This seemed to be the sound of a shotgun and I was surprised ... This was followed shortly by a loud bang on my door ... when I opened the door Andrew pushed a shotgun against my forehead. He placed the muzzle of the shotgun against my forehead, pushing me back into the room. The impact of the shotgun of my forehead caused a slight wound. I grabbed the barrel of the gun, forcing it to point downwards. With my body I pushed Andrew against the wall and then out on to the landing. I cried 'No, no, Andrew', and he said 'Yes'. He had a terrifying look in his eye and I knew he wanted to kill me. I was screaming 'Help me, help me' and these cries must have attracted Andrew Muggleton ... who immediately came to help me. In the course of the struggle Andrew never let go of the gun and fired it. The shots were directed at the wall. The atmosphere was filled with smoke. The sound of the gun going off filled me with terror. I recall that Andrew Muggleton managed to wrench the gun from Robinson's hands and this was thrown through the bannister railings ... With the gun having been taken from him, he tried to grasp me by the neck with his hands, but I managed to break free and run downstairs ...

Andrew Robinson's account of the incident in a statement to the police stated:

I had been informed by a doctor that when other doctors that he knew had committed suicide they had always used a gun and I saw that as the only effective means of killing myself if the depression did not cease. My intention was to have the gun stationed in my room and when in a fit of depression to use it on myself. However, when I applied for a shotgun certificate to enable me to purchase one, my application was rejected. I realised that the only way I should be able to obtain a gun was by borrowing or theft ... it was often impracticable for me to commit suicide. Thus in a bad state of depression I required some stimulus to draw me to the act of suicide. I could only think of [Miss B.] as the excuse if my fits of malice were uncommon [sic]. I had thought on certain occasions when I was shocked of hurting [Miss B.] and then doing away with myself. I had been extremely depressed yesterday. I realised that I was extremely ill even if for much I was virtually back to normal ... At about half past one to quarter to two this afternoon I had a vague idea of committing suicide. I got drunk and in the absence of my friend Tony Unsworth ... I took his gun and hid it by the stream at the College ... I thought that I had better do something at that moment to kill myself, my thoughts automatically turned to [Miss B.]. I hoped to inspire in her a savage reaction and frighten her and to hurt her, thus making my suicide inevitable ... When Tony and John approached me ... I ... fled. I then fired the gun at the base of a sapling to find out how it worked. After my friends fled I ran up to [Miss B.'s] room and not fully certain of my intentions, but with the thought of seriously hurting her and killing myself ... I violently tried to force an entrance into [Miss B.'s] room but she repelled me and prevented me from shooting her ... the violence of her rebuff forced an instant reaction of malice from me, and when I tried to shoot her she was assisted by a male student who wrestled the gun off me. As we wrestled for possession of the gun it fired ... I ... returned to [Miss B.'s] room, where in annoyance and malice I threw her books out of the window and smashed her plants ... In my depression my intentions as far as [Miss B.] was concerned was as I couldn't hurt her mind was to hurt her mind through her body and scar her for life ...

Andrew Robinson was charged with (a) possession of a firearm with intent to endanger life; and (b) assault occasioning actual bodily harm. He might easily have faced the more serious criminal offence of attempted murder. He pleaded guilty to both charges at Cardiff Crown Court on 26 September 1978. A Hospital Order with a Restriction Order unlimited in time were made. Dr Tidmarsh gave evidence strongly advising committal indefinitely to Broadmoor 'as his illness and potential dangerousness are likely to be long-lasting'.

Irrespective of the label attached by the court to the criminal offence, the criminal event disclosed behaviour which, if repeated, could result in the death of someone. And so long as Andrew Robinson's mental illness persisted, danger lurked for anyone who crossed his path, particularly a young woman. The risk of danger to anyone hung over him – at least when he was psychotic – like a brooding omnipresence. The murderous quality of that incident, clearly discernible from an examination of the police statements taken in preparation for the criminal trial, was consistently downgraded or devalued as the summaries of the event were handed down through the psychiatric services.

The earliest downgrading of the criminal event, following Andrew Robinson's conditional discharge from Broadmoor in April 1982, came in a letter of 4 October 1982 from Dr Nancy Pears to Dr Gerry Conway, requesting the latter to take over Andrew's care and treatment. She wrote:

> In the summer term Andrew landed up in prison, having threatened a girl whom he had known (and probably been teased by) with a shotgun. No damage was done, eventually Andrew was transferred to Broadmoor ...

Four years later, on 30 April 1986, Andrew's supervising officer, Steven Driscoll, wrote in his report to the MHRT that Andrew during the summer term of 1978 'became very emotionally disturbed and threatened his girlfriend with a shotgun'. In a similar vein, Dr Conway's report of 10 June 1986 to the MHRT in advocating the removal of the restriction order stated: 'While at this University, he formed a romantic liaison with a woman some six years his senior and when this relationship broke up, he is alleged to have gone to her room with a shot gun.'

Contemporaneously, the clinical note on Andrew's compulsory admission on 25 April 1986 stated: 'Summer 1978 – imprisoned having threatened girl-friend with shotgun' – no doubt gleaned exclusively from Andrew himself.

By contrast, the statement of May 1986 by the Home Secretary for the consideration of the Tribunal had, in summary form, accurately reflected the essence of the 1978 offence, thus:

> The circumstances of the offences were that on the afternoon of 3

June 1978 at Lampeter University Mr Robinson illegally acquired a
shotgun from a fellow student's room and discharged two shots; one
in the campus grounds, the other inside a building whilst struggling
with a female student with whom he had had a sexual relationship
and whom he admitted he had intended to maim.

Shortly after discharge from Moorhaven Hospital on 25 September
1986 Dr Conway's SHO wrote in his discharge summary, dated 2
October 1986, about the 1978 incident as follows:

> Events following the overdose are somewhat hazy but it seemed that
> his friends were extremely anxious at his having taken an overdose
> because of his depression and they were worried about his mental
> state and felt that this would be improved if he got back together
> with his girlfriend. To this end they arranged for the girl to say that
> she didn't feel as badly about him as she had previously said, that
> in fact things weren't as bad as he thought. When Andrew found this
> was not the case he reacted extremely strongly, details are unclear,
> but it seems that he had been drinking and then borrowed a friend's
> shot gun and threatened the girlfriend with this ...

Following Andrew Robinson's short admission in November 1986
to Exminster Hospital, Dr Moss's SHO, Dr Moira Cullen, in her
discharge summary of 28 November 1986 stated:

> He was very reluctant to talk about the following events that led up
> to his admission to Broadmoor, but they appear to have involved
> Andrew pulling a shotgun on his girlfriend, who is the mother of his
> child, Ben ...

This conflation of two completely discrete episodes, five or six years
apart, was candidly acknowledged at the Inquiry by Dr Cullen who
explained that the mix-up was the result of information she had
received, probably in her interview with Andrew Robinson.

A partial restoration of the true account of the 1978 incident was
achieved in a letter to Dr Moss from Dr Patrick Gallwey, Andrew's
RMO at the Butler Clinic in 1989. After Dr Gallwey's assessment
for Andrew's admission to the Butler Clinic, he wrote, on 10
February 1989:

> He then built up a deep sense of grudge [for Miss B.] which, from
> previous reports emerges as the development of a paranoid psychosis
> in which she was central to a paranoid delusion of attempting to
> destroy him. He went into her room with a loaded shotgun, which
> went off in the struggle. He maintains now that he had no intention

of hurting her, although it seems from previous records that he was actively psychotic and she could very easily have been killed.

Dr Moss's report for the Health Authority in respect of the review of the Guardianship Order in May 1989 was unhelpfully laconic in its description of the 1978 event. Even more laconic was his report to the MHRT on 16 August 1989. On 19 May 1989 he had said: 'During the summer of 1978, he [Andrew Robinson] became very emotionally disturbed, and threatened his girlfriend with a shotgun.' The August report to the MHRT said: 'On his recovery, he attempted to murder his ex-girlfriend using a shotgun.'

Much the same truncated version of the incident appeared in the discharge summary of 27 November 1989 by Dr Moss's SHO, Dr Cannizarro. He noted: '1978 – He overdosed following the breakup of a relationship and on recovery attempted to murder his ex-girlfriend using a shotgun.' This was repeated verbatim in a discharge summary of 24 July 1990, and again on 18 March 1991 by Dr Moss in his report to the MHRT. The same, one-sentence description of the ugly and worrying incident of 1978 appeared during Andrew's final admission to EMC in 1993. On 2 August 1993 in a letter from Dr McLaren to Dr Gillespie, asking him to assess Andrew Robinson for Watcombe Hall, it was stated: 'He took an overdose of medication following the break up of a relationship with a girl. On his recovery he attempted to murder this woman using a shotgun.'

Apart from the inaccuracies, not to say distortions of the 1978 incident, the excessively concise summaries, which could not be faulted as being inaccurate, can never be substitutes for a full appreciation of the nature and extent of the index offence.

We would go further than merely to advocate a handing down of the original description of the criminal event from one professional carer and transfer to another. As the patient progresses (and regresses) through the mental health system, there should go with him a chronology. A full chronology did ultimately emerge in the documentation supplied to the Inquiry by the Special Hospitals Service Authority when Andrew Robinson was committed to Broadmoor in October 1993. Dr T. Exworthy's psychiatric summary dated 8 March 1994, in the style devised by Dr Tidmarsh and his colleagues on the admission unit at Broadmoor, was enthusiastically acclaimed by all our witnesses as a model to be adopted in any future similar case. Those who subsequently have the patient under their care will know in sufficient detail the precise nature of the index offence, the record of later events relevant to the patient's mental disorder, and will be able to add to the chronology such material as is thought necessary for the up-to-date completion of the psychiatric history as the patient passes through mental health services.

VI. First Diagnosis of Schizophrenia

A psychiatrist is a person who treats disease with mental symptoms, not one who offers to transform the normally abrasive relations between men into a tedium of stultifying harmony.[*]

The gradual emergence of Andrew Robinsons's psychotic illness was in many ways characteristic. In October 1976, while studying economics in his first term at Lancaster University, he became preoccupied with the shape of his nose. A common-enough focus of dissatisfaction among young people, in most cases a preoccupation with the nasal configuration merely reflects a heightened personal vanity, often partly based on a realistic appreciation of one's own conventional facial attractiveness compared with others of the same age. In a small proportion of cases, however, the nose becomes the focus of obsessive dissatisfaction, being blamed for all perceived personal failings and social difficulties; in a yet smaller proportion this so-called 'dysmorphophobia' reflects delusional beliefs which are diagnostic pointers to a psychotic illness in which the beliefs are usually of a bizarre nature. We do not know whether the beliefs in Andrew Robinson's case in the early days were bizarre or not. The likelihood is that he did not express obvious delusional beliefs, since he was able in the following winter vacation to convince a plastic surgeon in London to operate on his nose. He was dissatisfied with the results of surgery. He has remained so ever since, and from time to time has continued to blame the shape of his nose for his failure to form good relationships with women.

He never returned to Lancaster University. After summer 1977, when he worked in a French camp site, he went to St David's College, Lampeter at the University of Wales, to read French. Within a few short weeks his mental state was deteriorating rapidly. As we have seen in Chapter V above, the following year, in August 1978, Dr Tidmarsh in his report to the court described this period of Andrew Robinson's life, based on Andrew's own account, as characterised by obsessive preoccupation with Miss B.,

---

[*] Henry Miller, 'The Abuse of Psychiatry' *Encounter* 34 (S) (1970), pp. 24-31.

culminating in an overdose of aspirin and paracetamol and his admission to the psychiatric unit at West Wales General Hospital. Andrew Robinson returned home to Devon after this episode, which was described by his father during our Inquiry as 'very alarming' for his family. His parents until then had no inkling of the torment their son was suffering, and had been inclined to attribute his worries about his nose to understandable 'adolescent nonsense'. On his return to Lampeter for his second term, he attended a clinical psychologist, perhaps three times, for psychotherapy, but his depression and fixation on Miss B. continued. At some point during this term he cut his wrists, one wrist requiring sutures, and sought further surgery on his nose, which was subsequently carried out in the Easter vacation, without any benefit as far as he was concerned.

Until the index offence, there had been no overt, unequivocal symptoms of psychosis. Dr Edwards, consultant psychiatrist at Glangwili, had concluded that Andrew Robinson was suffering from a 'personality disorder'. After the index offence, however, the nature and extent of his serious mental illness became clear. Dr Alan Capstick, consultant psychiatrist at Whitchurch Hospital, Cardiff, examined Andrew Robinson twice while he was in Cardiff Prison awaiting trial, in order to prepare a report on Andrew's fitness to plead and give an opinion on his psychiatric condition. Dr Capstick's opinion was that Andrew was suffering from paranoid schizophrenia; he judged that the illness had been developing insidiously for the past three years. This view was shared by Dr Denis Power, Senior Medical Officer at Cardiff Prison, an honorary consultant psychiatrist at the University of Wales, in his report to the Department of Health of 26 July 1978, recommending a Hospital Order and placement in a Special Hospital.

Dr Power's recommendation resulted in an assessment on 29 August 1978 by Dr David Tidmarsh, consultant psychiatrist at Broadmoor Hospital, who concurred with the diagnosis of schizophrenia and wrote:

> I strongly advise a Section 60 [Mental Health Act] with a restriction order under Section 65 without limit of time as his illness and potential dangerousness are likely to be long lasting.

It must be conceded, however, that none of these three psychiatrists' reports includes descriptions of symptoms which would be regarded as pathognomic of the diagnosis of schizophrenia. Indeed,

Dr Tidmarsh points out in this report that, while Andrew Robinson believed Miss B. was an evil influence on others, 'I was unable to elicit any more grandiose delusions, hallucinations or ideas of reference.' He did, however, regard his idea about his nose as a delusion. Andrew had been receiving substantial doses of neuroleptic medication while in prison, which may well have obscured any clear symptoms. Nevertheless, in the light of later queries about the diagnosis, it is important to note that in these experts' reports no 'first-rank symptoms' of schizophrenia were described.

Schneider,[1] an American psychiatrist, has distinguished a set of symptoms which in the absence of somatic illness point to a decisive clinical diagnosis of schizophrenia; these are (a) audible thoughts, voices heard arguing, voices heard commenting on one's actions; (b) the experience of influences playing on the body (somatic passivity experiences); (c) thought-withdrawal and other interferences with thoughts; (d) diffusion of thought, delusional perception; and (e) an experience that emotions, impulses and volitional acts are the work of, or influenced by, others. While Mellor's later study[2] demonstrated that these symptoms were not found universally in people with unequivocal diagnoses of schizophrenia (and in recent years less emphasis has been given to them as necessary for the diagnosis), they remain important pointers and are actively sought during mental state examination. The failure of these three psychiatrists to document any first-rank symptoms might well raise a query in the mind of a later reader that too much had been read into a number of 'overvalued' ideas. There is, however, one convincing description of delusions of control in the medical report of Cardiff Prison Medical Officer, Dr B.W. Oakley, dated 6 September 1978, in support of the Hospital Order:

> He was deluded that the female student had the mind of the devil and she was the source of evil power and propagated evil. He was deluded in that he thought she had the power to make him and other male students act corruptly by forcing them to damage her mind or sexually assault her. He experienced an irresistible compulsion to shoot her, over which he had no control.

Dr Oakley may have had an advantage over his psychiatric colleagues of being the generalist medical officer carrying out

---

[1] Schneider, K., *Clinical Psychopathology*. Grune and Stratton, New York (1939).
[2] Mellor, C.S., 'First rank symptons of schizophrenia'. *British Journal of Psychiatry* (1970), 117, 15-24.

routine prison medical work, and probably therefore examined Andrew Robinson during the early weeks of his remand, before medication had modified his beliefs.

On 26 September 1978 Andrew Robinson was committed to Broadmoor Hospital by means of a Hospital Order with restriction (without limit of time) under Sections 60 and 65 of the Mental Health Act 1959, where he came under the care of Dr Edgar Udwin. Dr Udwin never had any doubts about the diagnosis, describing his patient, in a letter to a colleague in South Africa, dated 4 June 1980, as 'manifestly schizophrenic', although he felt that there was a strong 'affective', that is mood-related, component to the disorder. Shortly after admission Andrew Robinson was 'extremely excitable, emotionally labile and ready to talk endlessly about his central delusion, which was the shape of his nose which he felt had affected not only his appearance and his mental state but also his bodily functioning'.

Dr Udwin told us that during his early days at Broadmoor Andrew Robinson was displaying 'a cocktail, shall we say, of symptomatology which in the view of Dr Tidmarsh and myself was dominated by the fact that he was psychotic'. His view was supported by the report in October 1980 of the Principal Psychologist at Broadmoor, Tony Black. In Dr Udwin's view, Andrew Robinson's severely disordered personality was part and parcel of the dominant mental illness, and a diagnosis of personality or psychopathic disorder was 'something other again and not relevant in this context'.

The diagnosis of schizophrenia was thus clearly established in 1978. The international systems of diagnosis and classification of psychiatric disorders, used for the purposes of research and for compiling comparative international statistical data, are now rooted in the principle of a hierarchy of diagnosis in which specific psychotic symptoms take precedence in the allocation of diagnosis over symptoms of mood or other non-specific symptoms of behaviour or personality disturbance. Computerised diagnostic systems, which are now considered essential tools of psychiatric epidemiology, are explicitly designed to reflect this approach.[3] Once a person has exhibited specific symptoms of schizophrenia over a prolonged period of months or years, subsequent symptoms of disturbance in

---

[3] Wing, J.K., Cooper, J.E., Sartorius, N., *The Measurement and Classification of Psychiatric Disorders.* Cambridge University Press, London (1974).

personal relationships can be understood in terms of the psychotic illness and do not require a separate or distinct diagnosis of 'personality disorder'. To label them as such is indeed to imply that the schizophrenia never existed. As we shall see later, Andrew Robinson's care was significantly affected by the diagnosis of schizophrenia being 'overturned', or 'sidelined', later in his career.

VII. Thirty Months at Broadmoor, September 1978 – July 1981

> In many cases an individual, in pursuing a legitimate object, neces-
> sarily and therefore legitimately causes pain or loss to others, or
> intercepts a good which they had a reasonable hope of obtaining.
> Such oppositions of interest between individuals often arise from bad
> social institutions but are unavoidable while those institutions last;
> and some would be unavoidable under any institutions.[*]

Andrew Robinson's stay in Broadmoor was comparatively short –
just three months short of three years – whereas the average stay
for patients was at that time about six years. From the accounts of
both his RMO, Dr Edgar Udwin, and his family, it was a successful
admission. His psychotic illness markedly improved with neuroleptic medication; by 1980 Dr Udwin described him as 'currently well
controlled on medication although by no means in full remission.
He is no way violent and I think could be controlled, providing he
remains on injectable medication, in the community, although the
possibility of relapses has to be considered.' Throughout his stay in
Broadmoor there was no hint of aggression or violence in either his
deeds or his thoughts, as recorded by mental state examination in
the psychologist's reports. As Dr Udwin told us 'He was admitted
non-violent, remained non-violent throughout and he was discharged non-violent'.

By the time of his transfer to Exe Vale Hospital in July 1981
Andrew Robinson had begun to develop some insight into the
delusional nature of his worries about his physical appearance. He
was, however, throughout his stay in Broadmoor, troubled by
extrapyramidal side-effects of the medication and continued to
complain of the unwanted effects whenever he had been on regular
medication, a significant and understandable factor in his reluctance to continue it.

In answer to Mr Thorold's question, 'How did he [Andrew] take
to being in Broadmoor?' his father told us: 'At the time he took to

[*] John Stuart Mill, 'Applications', in *On Liberty* (1859), Penguin Classics (1985),
ch. V, pp. 163-4.

it very well, or seemed to us to take to it very well', and commented: 'He was in the workshops every day, in the printing department, for several hours. He read for a qualification in electronics, for which he got some certificate. He seemed on the whole to have – it was one of the best times of the whole period, really, when he was there, in some ways.'

Dr Udwin invested a good deal of effort in trying to arrange for Andrew to be transferred to psychiatric care in hospital in South Africa, at the request of his parents who were hoping at that time to settle there on a permanent basis, and were living in Durban during the early part of 1981. The warm and helpful letters exchanged between Dr Udwin and the Rev. Peter Robinson give the reader the impression that the relationship was one of mutual trust and respect between the consultant and his patient's nearest relatives. They seemed to have established a rapport which was rarely achieved by his later psychiatrists. In the event, Andrew Robinson's parents returned to live in Devon. The careful plans for Andrew's care and treatment in South Africa were abortive.

These contemporaneous observations, that he settled well at Broadmoor, were not mirrored after his discharge by Andrew's own retrospective opinions. He certainly gave Dr Conway the impression that his time in Broadmoor had been a terrible experience and that many of his subsequent difficulties originated at Broadmoor. Dr Conway told us: 'He was very hurt by Broadmoor and he felt that it had changed him and damaged him. He was afraid of Broadmoor, I think that would be a better way of putting it. He was very much afraid of Broadmoor and of ever being in a position of being sent back there.' Andrew Robinson's later perception of his days at Broadmoor was coloured by frank delusional ideas that he had been 'irradiated' there, and that Dr Udwin continued to control his mind. His own account of his Broadmoor years, however, seems to have been accepted uncritically by Dr Conway, who was convinced that Andrew's horror of Broadmoor would act as an effective deterrent to future wrong-doing. In his report for the MHRT in 1986, at which he recommended Andrew Robinson's discharge, he wrote 'I feel that Mr Robinson has been so distressed by his experiences at Broadmoor that he would be afraid to embark on any violent behaviour for fear of being sent back to prison or indeed to Broadmoor Hospital'. He might have considered Andrew's attitude to Broadmoor unhealthily overvalued, had he had the benefit of reading the clinical notes and taking the Rev. and Mrs Robinson's opinions into account.

It may well be true of course that the kind of regime at Broadmoor in which Andrew Robinson was treated was experienced by him as over-restrictive and frustrating, and this would not necessarily have been obvious to his RMO or to visitors. But it is important to note that when Dr Nancy Pears, consultant psychiatrist, and her clinical team visited Andrew at Broadmoor in March 1981, with a view to his transfer to Exe Vale Hospital, they were much impressed by what they observed. She wrote to Dr Udwin after the visit: '... a lot was gained [by the team] by seeing some of the ways in which you help your very difficult patients and I hope some of it will rub off ... The positive approach of Broadmoor was most impressive.' Dr Udwin's view, expressed to us – and one we share – was that Andrew's period at Broadmoor was successful and enabled him to be considered for an early conditional discharge to an open unit.

In Dr Udwin's opinion, two factors would be crucial in maintaining Andrew Robinson in the community – medication and supervision:

> One has a number of things to consider, whether one is considering a conditional discharge or even a transfer to another hospital, and top of the list, I think, comes something you can put a stroke next to. It is cooperation-cum-supervisability. If a man is going out on discharge one wants to know that he is going to accept and cooperate with supervision, that he sees the need for a number of things, including the conditions you lay down, and that very much puts medication at the top of the list. At the same time on a transfer one has to consider and consult with the receiving consultant about the available facilities at his hospital, his confidence in taking on such a case ...

In October 1980, Dr Udwin assessed Andrew's future likelihood of becoming dangerous as follows:

> Currently one can confidently predict that the likelihood of aggression unless similar circumstances arose would be entirely negligible. As regards the recurrence of the same delusional situation in the face of another unfortunate relationship with a female, the view can be taken that the hazards are much reduced by the fact that his condition is known and that he is under the control of medication.

He added to that report for us:

I think that I was perhaps a bit slipshod in my writing of this report because 'under the control of medication' should have been followed by 'and supervision'. The combination of those two would minimise risks but I point out, as I pointed out before, that no one is infallible and errors can occur no matter how close the supervision. It is a reduction of risks to the absolute minimum, [to which we would add 'the irreducible minimum'].

When asked directly by one of us, whether at the time of Andrew's conditional discharge Dr Udwin expected him to continue supervision and medication in perpetuity, he answered: 'Certainly for many years. It is hard to say in perpetuity.' The Chairman interjected 'Indefinitely?', to which Dr Udwin responded 'Indefinitely'. He told us, furthermore, that had he been asked for an opinion at the time, that he would have recommended to the Mental Health Review Tribunal in 1986 that the conditional discharge arrangements should remain in place for the foreseeable future.

Andrew Robinson left Broadmoor for Exe Vale Hospital on 15 July 1981, his future looking infinitely brighter than many would have predicted on his admission in 1978.

VIII. The Shadow Begins to Fall: Post-Broadmoor Pattern of Life

It is a distinguishing characteristic of the Erewhonians that when they profess themselves to be quite certain about any matter, and avow it as a base on which they are to build a system of practice, they seldom quite believe in it. If they smell a rat about the precepts of a cherished institution, they will always stop their noses to it if they can.*

The preparation for Andrew Robinson's transfer from Broadmoor to the Exe Vale Hospital in Exeter was carefully arranged between Dr Udwin and Dr Pears. In March 1981 Dr Pears was asked whether she would agree to assess and accept Andrew Robinson as a catchment-area patient for a short period before he emigrated to South Africa. On 25 March 1981, Dr Pears, after having assessed Andrew, wrote: 'I agree with you that Andrew Robinson is now ready for transfer to an open mental hospital, as he is not now violent.' Dr Pears' understanding was that Andrew would be admitted to Exe Vale for a period of two months prior to transfer to South Africa. He was transferred on 15 July 1981.

The notes relating to Andrew's period at Exe Vale Hospital were not available to the Inquiry, but accounts of his progress appear in letters from Dr Pears and to the Home Office, Dr Udwin and Dr Conway. It appears that Andrew made 'very good progress' and by November 1981 was 'now virtually free of psychotic signs and symptoms'. Arrangements for his transfer to South Africa dragged on for months without the emigration being effected. Ultimately, the exercise was abandoned, Andrew's parents having by late 1981 returned to England.

By May 1982 Dr Pears was considering conditional discharge of Andrew from hospital to the community in this country. Her letter to the Home Office requested agreement in principle to conditional discharge and carried the opinion that 'he [Andrew Robinson] needs to continue (medication) indefinitely. So long as his illness remains controlled and he receives sufficient emotional support

---

* Samuel Butler, *Erewhon*, ch. XVIII.

and supervision from trained professionals, I do not consider there to be any unacceptable risk of violent behaviour.' The theme of continued medication under supervision was reiterated by all the professionals, with the notable exception of Dr Conway.

Dr Pears wrote to Dr Conway asking him if he would consider taking over Andrew's care, were he to be conditionally discharged, which would mean that Andrew would return to live with his parents, locating him within Dr Conway's catchment area. On 27 November 1981, Dr Conway interviewed Andrew and his parents, and agreed to provide medical supervision on a 4-6 weekly outpatient basis.

The Home Office agreed on 27 January 1983 to Andrew's conditional discharge from section 65 of the Mental Health Act 1959, under the supervision of Dr Conway and social worker, Mr Hooper. On 24 February 1983 Dr Conway became the RMO for Andrew, with Mr Hooper his supervising officer under the conditional discharge.

Under the 1959 Mental Health Act (as indeed under the 1983 Act) the RMO had certain responsibilities for restricted patients on conditional discharge. Those included furnishing the Home Office with quarterly reports, with information about the patient's current mental state, his dangerousness, his level of functioning and his compliance with treatment. The Home Office also required the RMO to notify it of any changes in behaviour or circumstances that might have a bearing on the level of risk the patient posed, either to himself or others. It is clear to us that Dr Conway was fully aware of these requirements.

During 1982 Andrew continued to live with his parents, to attend outpatient appointments with Dr Conway approximately six-weekly, and to see Mr Hooper at similar intervals. He had a relationship with a fellow patient who gave birth to their son in May 1983, but they never lived together as a family unit. Throughout this period the reports to the Home Office are largely reassuring, with the only concerns being raised, without a great deal of emphasis, by Mr Hooper. In July 1983 Mr Hooper wrote: 'His expressed attitude to women does give me some slight cause for concern, in that he is very fixed in the view that they can only respect someone who dominates them.' In August 1983 Mr Hooper's report makes reference to Andrew Robinson's capacity to 'tease and provoke' his girlfriend, but it also states 'he remains as well as I have seen him'. In December 1983 reference is made to

Andrew's writing: 'He tells me most of his time is taken up with writing and re-writing his book, but the more I hear of it the more it appears to be somewhat self-indulgent.' Mr Hooper acknowledged to us that at this stage he felt that 'the writing of the book was virtually obsessional'.

As early as July 1983 Andrew was indicating that he would like to move out of his parents' home to more independent accommodation. This theme continued, and by 15 May 1984 arrangements were in place for him to move to his own flat in Exeter, with the responsibility for medical supervision passing to Dr Tillett, and social work supervision to Mr Langley-Smith. By early August 1984 living in Exeter had proved unsuccessful and Andrew returned once more to live with his parents, reverting to the care of Dr Conway and Mr Hooper.

Two weeks after his return, a family friend, Lady Rashleigh, wrote to Dr Conway expressing her concerns about Andrew's continuing preoccupation with his nose and his need for cosmetic surgery. This was not viewed by Dr Conway, he told us, as having any 'pathological significance'.

Over the following months Andrew remained concerned about his nose, and made a further appointment with a plastic surgeon in December. The same family friend again wrote to Dr Conway, as did Andrew's GP Dr Steggles, informing him of Andrew's continued preoccupation. Dr Conway's report to the Home Office of 24 January 1985 acknowledged that Andrew's nose was an issue for him, but concludes: 'I was quite satisfied ... with his clinical presentation and do not see him as being in any way deranged mentally.' Three weeks previously, Mr Hooper had written to Dr Conway expressing various concerns. In the letter he reported: 'During the interview he [Andrew Robinson] got quite animated and spoke of feeling very depressed and how this depression was lifted in the past by violent action.' Dr Conway told us that he did not think 'this raised alarm bells at the time'. Again, from oral evidence given by Mr Hooper, it is clear that little effective consultation took place between Dr Conway and other professionals; hence Mr Hooper's concerns would not have been promoted in any regular multi-disciplinary forum in which the issue could be explored.

In March 1985 Dr Conway stopped Andrew's medication. The notes contain no explanation for this course of action; nor could Dr Conway recount to us what his reasons had been for discontinuing medication. At the time, Dr Conway's diagnosis of Andrew was one of personality disorder as opposed to the diagnosis of schizophrenia that had been made by all RMOs since Andrew's admission to Broadmoor in 1978.

In April 1985 Mr Hooper ceased to be Andrew's social worker and the role was taken on by Mr Gleeson. In July 1985 Andrew moved with his parents to Stoke Fleming. By 6 August 1985 Andrew's father was sufficiently concerned about his son to write to Dr Conway. Andrew was described as 'depressed, extremely restless and very aggressive and belligerent ...'. The letter continued: 'My wife ... feel(s) that he should be on some medication.' There is no evidence from the notes that this letter prompted a reassessment of Andrew's treatment regime, nor in oral evidence could Dr Conway confirm whether any such reassessment had occurred. On 8 August Dr Conway saw Andrew in outpatients, and reported to the Home Office: 'I can find no evidence of any schizophrenic process or indeed any evidence of mental illness'.

On 23 August 1985 Dr Conway was sent a letter of complaint from Lady Rashleigh with whom Andrew was now living. The complaint was about the approach of the social worker who was supervising Andrew. Mr Hooper, the principal social worker, investigated the matter and on 12 September wrote to Dr Conway advising against changing the social worker, as the complainant had requested. On 25 September 1985 Dr Conway was sent a letter from the social worker involved, reporting concerns expressed by Lady Rashleigh that 'Andrew ... has become verbally aggressive and abusive to members of her family'. He further requested that a case conference be arranged as a matter of urgency. There is no evidence of any response to this letter. There is, however, a report to the Home Office, dated 11 October 1985, in which Dr Conway noted: 'He did appear rather more anxious than previously and it would seem that this is due to a difference of opinion which he had with his parents.' It further went on to request support for a change of social worker. In November 1985 Mr Driscoll took over from Mr Gleeson as Andrew's supervising social worker.

In taking over this role, Mr Driscoll, at Andrew's insistence, did not look at any hospital notes before taking a history from him. In Mr Driscoll's estimation this enabled him to build a good rapport with Andrew. Mr Driscoll told us that the history which he obtained from Andrew tallied with the information on file in matters of substance, although there were areas where there was a difference of interpretation.

The first report that Mr Driscoll sent to the Home Office, dated 17 December 1985, stated: 'At the moment I have no obvious cause for concern.' This was followed by a further report on 17 March 1985, in which Mr Driscoll wrote about being 'rather concerned about Andrew during my interview with him ... It was all somewhat bizarre and difficult to follow.' This was in conflict with the report submitted by Dr Conway on 18 February which stated: 'I still remain of the firm conviction that this man is not mentally ill as such at the present time.' This view was held, despite the receipt of a letter dated 27 January 1986 that was sent by Andrew's current landlady, Mrs Quiterio. She wrote to Dr Conway with an account of a very disturbed and disturbing night with Andrew during which he rushed downstairs and handed her a knife in the presence of her other residents, and played a tape of a conversation with Lady Rashleigh. He appeared to be extremely confused and distressed. She explained her reason for writing thus: 'We are very concerned, not only for the danger that Andrew might be to himself, but also, ... of what danger ... he might be to our family and other boarders. He seems harmless enough, but the very fact that he bought this knife either suggests he was considering suicide, or it was just a dramatic attempt to get attention from us all ... I would be grateful if you could act upon this letter and take whatever action you think necessary.' On 29 January 1986 Dr Conway wrote back to the landlady thanking her for her concern, but he did not see Andrew again until 17 February 1986; the relevant entry in the medical notes makes no reference to Andrew's mental state, nor to the concern raised by the landlady.

Further concerns about Andrew's condition were raised by Mr Driscoll in his report to the Home Office of 18 March 1986, as quoted above, and by Andrew's father in a letter to Dr Conway dated 1 April 1986 that stated: 'In my opinion, and that of many others, he is very ill and should be receiving medication, possibly in hospital ...'

In his report to the Home Office on 22 April 1986, Dr Conway conceded that all was not well. Andrew had failed to keep his outpatient appointment, and further reports that he was causing concern had been received from the family friend who thought that Andrew 'seemed to be very troubled with deluded ideas and felt that various messages were being conveyed to him in the newspapers in some sort of code'. In Dr Conway's view, 'this patient's condition has clearly regressed since I saw him last and the indications as described ... are somewhat suggestive of a relapsing paranoid illness'. His report ended:

> I propose to establish whether I can arrange for a social worker to visit him in the very near future to determine whether he could be encouraged to come back and see me, with a view to resumption of treatment; whether it will prove necessary to invoke a section of the 1983 Mental Health Act will depend largely on his condition and presentation at the time of interview with the social worker visiting him.

On 25 April 1986 Andrew was compulsorily admitted to Moorhaven Hospital on section 3 of the Mental Health Act 1983. The admission was precipitated by 'repeated calls from (the family friend) and the police in Stoke Fleming' to the duty social work team through whom a Mental Health Act assessment was arranged. Dr Conway was not involved in the admission and did not see him until 30 April 1986. When he did review the case, he stopped the medication, Stelazine and Melleril, that had been prescribed on admission. The rationale for this discontinuation is unclear and remained unexplained before us.

Andrew remained in Moorhaven until 25 September 1986, having been converted into an informal patient on 17 September. During his inpatient stay he continued to be off all medication. His behaviour at times gave significant concern to a range of staff involved in his care. There are in the medical, social work and nursing notes accounts of several episodes that made staff feel uneasy. On 6 May Dr Conway's secretary was forced to lock herself in her office. On 29 May Dr Hambly made an entry in the notes about a telephone conversation he had had with Andrew's ex-girlfriend, who told him that 'Andrew has been very abusive to her. He has grabbed her around the neck on one occasion in an argument. She ... feels harassed by him.' On 30 May it was reported that 'Steve Driscoll ... reports extreme anxieties about Andrew's ability to control himself when outside hospital. He is concerned that Andrew is a risk to others in his state of mind off treatment.' On 4 June 1986 an entry in the nursing notes recorded: 'Andrew became quite foul-mouthed and abusive towards myself at tea time this evening. Using foul language he began shouting personal sexual questions, pointed at me, but shouted up and down the ward.' The entry continued in that vein. Entries on 5, 7 and 9 June added to the emerging picture of Andrew having periods of disturbed behaviour with a strong paranoid flavour.

This is further reflected in a report from the Principal Clinical Psychologist, dated 13 June 1986, that concluded: 'Although I found no evidence of formal thought disorder, it seemed clear to me that Mr Robinson is preoccupied with thoughts of a persecutory and paranoid nature, which he acknowledges but insists on maintaining.' On 22 June 1986 there was a further nursing note that read: 'Awoke in angry mood. It is not possible to reason with Andrew this morning as he is so angry and abusive, continually storming up and down corridor using foul language, coming into office making sweeping statements such as "Dr Conway and Steve Driscoll are F-up my life and are murderers" etc etc. Conversation, such as it is, is largely of a sexual nature: how many suicides does Dr Conway need per year to get sexual gratification? Continually asking personal questions of a sexual nature. Threw cup of coffee over corridor and walls.' When we asked whether such an account in the context of the other material mentioned had led Dr Conway to reconsider his diagnosis of personality disorder, he felt it had not, and continued: 'It is just he got out of bed the wrong side that particular day.'

On 29 June 1986 the nursing notes referred to Andrew: 'Apparently bothering family of girl he attempted to shoot by telephone constantly.' That was the start of a four-week period in which there were regular records in both nursing and medical notes of Andrew's activities in trying to contact witnesses from his original trial. Complaints about his activities were received from the police in Barnstaple and in the Isle of Wight, from medical staff at Broadmoor and from an individual who was at college with Andrew and who was concerned about his own safety. These were quite disturbing attempts to harass.

Running through this period there were also accounts of frequent angry outbursts, often with a paranoid flavour. Despite the behavioural disturbance that he was exhibiting, Andrew was granted 10 days' leave of absence by Dr Conway on 15 August 1986. He was still on no medication. On 27 August a further report made no mention of Andrew's attempts to contact the trial witnesses, an omission for which Dr Conway could offer no explanation when he appeared before us. The report did state that 'since the time of admission ... there has been no untoward behaviour or any evidence of aggression or violent propensity'. When we asked how he came to write this, in the light of the recorded instances of violent behaviour, Dr Conway replied: 'I don't know. I can't explain that. I presume I was swayed by the fact he hadn't actually attacked anybody or hurt anybody.' Dr Conway's report also noted that 'Female nurses are unanimous in stating that they have never felt in any way threatened and intimidated by him', and yet four days before the Tribunal an entry in the nursing notes reports:

> Andrew seemed to settle after highly charged outbursts this morning but by mid-afternoon was continuing to sound persecuted and distraught about Tribunals, Courts, Nazis etc. obviously as angry towards us, system.

And later in the same notes:

> Close to striking me.

At this time Andrew's application, made earlier in 1986, for a Mental Health Review Tribunal was imminent. We describe the events before and at the hearing in Chapter IX. Both Dr Conway and Mr Driscoll submitted reports to the Tribunal. While Mr Driscoll's view at the time of the Tribunal was that the conditional discharge should remain, Dr Conway submitted a report, dated 10 June 1986, with a supplementary report written on 15 September 1986. Strongly advocating an absolute discharge, which was at least consistent with his termination of the section 3 order at the time of the Tribunal, these reports repeated Dr Conway's view that Andrew Robinson was not suffering from paranoid schizophrenia, and that he did not represent any threat to the public. When asked in oral evidence whether he now felt that his reports gave the Tribunal 'a fair and accurate reflection', Dr Conway conceded 'possibly not'. This he expanded: 'He would appear to have been – from the other references – rather more paranoid than I had led them to believe.' Again, when asked about his reports: 'Do you think, looking back on the notes, that you have minimised incidents of aggression, be it physical or verbal, on the part of Andrew', Dr Conway conceded: 'I may have underplayed them slightly, yes', but he could offer no explanation for this.

This period marks a significant turning point for Andrew Robinson. On discharge from Broadmoor in 1981 it was expected that he would continue on medication and be under supervision for a very long time, if not indefinitely. Dr Udwin, who had been his RMO in

Broadmoor, affirmed to us that, had he given evidence at the Tribunal in 1986, he would have supported the continuance of the conditional discharge. He was similarly unwavering in his belief that long-term medication was a key component of any treatment package for Andrew. This view, however, was not shared by Dr Conway, who chose to discontinue Andrew's medication in March 1985 and in April 1986 and was instrumental in securing Andrew's absolute discharge in September 1986. Several factors may have contributed to this outcome. Dr Conway seems to have worked very much as an individual consultant, rather than as a member of a multi-disciplinary team. His relationship with Andrew was key to the treatment pathway that he followed. The consultation with other professionals was minimal. There was ample evidence in the nursing notes of psychosis, notes which were regularly initialled by Dr Conway, indicating that he had read them; and yet he must have disregarded what he read.

Dr Conway appears to have accommodated Andrew's wishes, wherever possible, in an attempt to maintain Andrew's trust. This approach of advocacy for the patient, admirable in one sense, is an abandonment of professional standards which require objectivity and not collusion. Information from other sources – friends, family, other professionals – that was at variance with Dr Conway's personal experience of Andrew was either discounted or marginalised. Andrew Robinson was more than capable of maintaining a plausible façade for short periods, at will. Blind to Andrew's more psychotic aspects, and influenced by Andrew's distorted account of the maltreatment and injustice that he had supposedly suffered from psychiatric services and the criminal justice system, Dr Conway was led into misdiagnosis, flawed risk-assessment and highly selective communication with the Home Office. Together, these led to the abandonment of what Dr Udwin considered to be the indispensable conditions for safe community placement, namely continuing medication and supervision through the conditional discharge provisions.

Three main factors might have altered this disquieting outcome. First, the presence at Moorhaven of a strong and effective multi-disciplinary team might have challenged Dr Conway's perceptions and formulations about Andrew Robinson. There is plenty of evidence of clear-thinking by the professionals involved in Andrew's care, but there is a marked absence of any unified team approach. Additionally, formalised clinical supervision, had it been available to Dr Conway, might have encouraged him to reflect upon some of his attitudes and assumptions. It is a matter for concern that, while some mental health disciplines are making great strides in acknowledging the need, and setting-up systems for clinical supervision, psychiatry has not yet really got off the starting blocks.

Secondly – and this is a recurring theme throughout the mental health services handling Andrew Robinson – it is also possible that, had Dr Conway received full details of the index offence and subsequent treatment when he took over responsibility for Andrew, rather than relying on Andrew's distorted version, he might have approached assessment and treatment somewhat differently.

Thirdly, Dr Conway's lone advocacy for Andrew's discharge, unsupported by the otherwise unanimous view that, whatever the diagnosis of mental health, medication plus supervision would be absolutely necessary way beyond the five years out of Broadmoor, might not have prevailed had matters gone differently before the MHRT.

IX. Andrew Robinson, his RMO and the MHRT

> My experience has shown that in no case is it more difficult to elicit productive and reliable expert testimony than in cases that call on the knowledge and practice of psychiatry.*

The Mental Health Review Tribunal (MHRT) which sat on 19 September 1986 to hear Andrew Robinson's application to have the conditional discharge of 27 January 1983 converted into an absolute discharge – in effect to remove his liability to recall – was probably one of the earliest, if not *the* earliest occasion when an MHRT exercised its newly granted power under the Mental Health Act 1983 to make such an order. In describing and commenting on the circumstances whereby Andrew Robinson came to be finally released from any constraint under the provisions of the Mental Health Act, we are focusing our attention very much on the particular case. It is certainly not our function to perform a review of the mental health tribunal system, although we apprehend that such review is at present overdue, since we are aware of widespread criticism having been expressed in the specialist literature[1] and in some concerns on the part of Council on Tribunals in its last two reports.[2]

Some of the deficiencies that we have uncovered may or may not be relevant to the workings of the tribunals today, but we are conscious that the function of the MHRTs in September 1986 may project a very different picture to 1994 eyes. Anything we say about what went wrong in the decision-making process in September 1986 must not be taken as criticism of the MHRT which sat to hear Andrew Robinson's case. Indeed, we do not seek to question the

---

* Judge Bazelon, 'Psychiatrists and the Adversarial Process', 230 *Scientific American* 18 (June 1974). Judge Bazelon was a former judge of the US Court of Appeals for the District of Columbia and author of the Durham rule in 1954 on the criminal responsibility of the mentally disordered.

[1] E.g. Jill Peay, *Tribunals on Trial: a study of decision-making under the Mental Health Act 1983*. Clarendon Press (1989).

[2] Annual Report (1992-93) paras 2.60-2.63 and Annual Report (1993-94) paras 2.99-2.110.

correctness of the decision on the material then placed before the Tribunal members. We are not a court of appeal. With hindsight, enhanced by the uncovering of much documentary material which was unavailable to the MHRT, we do think that Andrew's liability to recall should have remained in existence, almost certainly indefinitely. We are even more confident in thinking that the three members of the MHRT would now, looking back on the case as it was presented to them and taking into account the same insights revealed to us in 1994, agree that they had come to a wrong decision. Justice plainly miscarried.

Our ability to review the case fully is in no small measure thanks to the members themselves, His Honour Judge Henry Palmer, Dr Derrick Ellis and Mr Thomas Dennis. We contacted Judge Palmer who readily responded, after consultation with his two colleagues, by directing the release of his own notes of the hearing and allowing us access to any other information. (The records were no longer in the possession of the MHRT administration.) Rule 21(5) of the Mental Health Review Tribunal Rules 1983 states that 'except in so far as the tribunal may direct, information about proceedings before the tribunal and the names of any persons concerned in the proceedings shall not be made public'. We did not stop to ask whether a direction to make the information about the proceedings on 19 September 1986 could be made years after the Tribunal has ceased to exercise its jurisdiction to hear and determine a patient's application (or consider a reference). The Rule would appear to relate to a power exercisable only during the duration of the proceedings before the MHRT, exceptionally to direct the disclosure of information. It may be that the extension of the power should be made explicit in any future amendments to the Rules.

Our ability to canvass the procedural steps taken by Judge Palmer and his colleagues was further augmented by a happy coincidence that Dr Ellis was, simultaneously to our oral hearings, attending at another tribunal at Torbay District General Hospital. He readily acceded to our invitation that he should give oral evidence and he did so, very helpfully, on the morning of 26 July 1994. Our fortune did not end with the oral testimony of Dr Ellis. With an assiduity of Gladstonian proportions, he had preserved the notes of every MHRT on which he had sat, a span of 35 years. The notes of his involvement in Andrew Robinson's case were invaluable in filling the spaces in the jigsaw puzzle – he was also a member of the Tribunal on two later occasions, first in December

1986, when Andrew appealed against a section 2 detention for assessment and, secondly, in September 1991, when he opposed the renewal of a Guardianship Order.

Background to the application for discharge

Andrew Robinson had been compulsorily admitted to Moorhaven Hospital in Plymouth on 25 April 1986 under section 3 of the Mental Health Act, suffering from schizophrenia. He was not recalled to hospital under the conditional discharge of 19 April 1982, although he could well have been. Dr Conway, who had been seeing Andrew as an outpatient ever since 1982, had become his RMO. Before his admission to Moorhaven, Andrew had applied to have his case considered by an MHRT. On 9 April 1986 the Home Office had written to Dr Conway asking for a report on Andrew Robinson's mental condition, seeking his views on the suitability or otherwise of the conditions presently attaching to Andrew's discharge. A similar letter was written to Andrew's supervising officer, Mr Steven Driscoll. By the time that both Dr Conway and Mr Driscoll sent in their reports, the section 3 admission of 25 April 1986 had been effected. During the coming months it was assumed that Andrew's application to the MHRT was directed to challenging the section 3 admission. In late August Dr Conway wrote to the Home Office indicating that he was minded to discharge the section 3 order and regrade Andrew as an informal patient. The section 3 order was, in practice, rescinded by Dr Conway on 17 September, by which time Andrew had purportedly withdrawn his application to the MHRT. Two days later the MHRT, in circumstances which we will describe in detail, removed the remnant of the restriction order, by way of an absolute discharge. Andrew Robinson discharged himself from Moorhaven as an informal patient on 25 September 1986.

The Home Office letter of 9 April 1986 had pointed out that under section 75 of the Mental Health Act 1983 the Tribunal had the power to vary the conditions attaching to the patient's discharge, or under sub-section 2(a) to direct that the restriction order should be terminated altogether. But that power was exercisable only if the conditionally discharged patient has not been recalled to hospital. Andrew had not been recalled, but had been readmitted under section 3. Thus the two controls on him – the conditional discharge and the section 3 compulsory admission – were running in parallel, although not in harness.

Given the two constraints on his freedom, a curiosity in the legislation arose. Section 41(3) provides that in the case of a restricted patient 'no application shall be made to a Mental Health Review Tribunal in respect of a patient under section 66 …'. Section 66(i)(b) provides that ordinarily an application can be made by a patient admitted to a hospital in pursuance of an application for admission for treatment – namely, section 3. Thus, until 17 September 1986, the MHRT could not lawfully entertain Andrew Robinson's application under section 75. Fortunately, although the Tribunal may not have realised the fact, on 19 September 1986 the jurisdictional encumbrance of section 41(3)(b) had fallen away. The Tribunal was properly constituted to do what it in fact did – namely, to consider discharging Andrew Robinson absolutely. Our understanding of the law is that the twin powers constitute an invalidity. The exclusion of the restricted patient's power to apply for a review – by virtue of section 41(3)(b) – is a clear violation of Article 5(4) of the European Convention on Human Rights. The reduction of the restricted patient's right to have a tribunal review appears to us also to be contrary to the spirit of the 1983 Act. The simple expedient would be to remove the barrier to a tribunal hearing in section 41(3)(b).

The hearing of 19 September 1986

Rule 11 of the Mental Health Review Tribunal Rules 1983 contains an odd provision. At any time – usually it is a few days – before the hearing of an application the medical member of the Tribunal 'shall examine the patient and take such other steps as he considers necessary to form an opinion of the patient's mental condition' – odd, because it is unclear whether what the medical member acquires by way of psychiatric examination of the patient constitutes part of the evidence, and can be disclosed to the parties, or whether it is merely part of the Tribunal's deliberative process. We do not need to add our twopennyworth to that debate, beyond pointing to a peculiar situation which arose in Andrew Robinson's case, calling at least for a review of Rule 11.

Four days before the hearing was due to take place, Dr Ellis visited Moorhaven Hospital to examine three patients, one of whom was Andrew Robinson. The nursing notes recorded that the previous day Andrew had expressed the wish not to see Dr Ellis, because he felt that any tribunal would in fact be biased against him. The entry for 15 September (the day of Dr Ellis's visit) stated: 'Burst into office this morning, during handover. Ranting and raving about MHRT, doctors and Dr Ellis's visit. Has *no* intention of seeing him or attending the tribunal. A few minutes later returned with a letter to give to Dr Ellis.' (The letter repeated Andrew's withdrawal, four months earlier, of his application.) In fact Andrew did attend the Tribunal on 19 September, but he had not been examined beforehand by Dr Ellis. Dr Ellis told us that he was handed the typed letter from Andrew – Dr Ellis has retained it to this day – and that was 'the sum total of my examination'. Dr Ellis said that this was the only occasion in his professional life on which he had been unable to examine a patient psychiatrically, to his complete satisfaction, before a tribunal hearing.

Rule 11, on the face of it, is mandatory – the medical member 'shall examine' the patient. The feature of the procedure in our legal system of one member of a tribunal acquiring information exclusively for himself, to be shared, second-hand, with his tribunal colleagues, with or without disclosure to the parties, is unusual. Any departure from normal procedures must be treated as having had special significance to the legislature. We wonder whether the Tribunal should or could have proceeded without compliance with Rule 11. Since MHRTs can, and do hear cases on reference (where the patient does not even apply for discharge from an order) it might be argued that a strict application of Rule 11 would be absurd. But the mere fact that the patient is not directly involved in his or her case – which is what happens in a case on reference – does not preclude the conduct of a psychiatric examination by the medical member in advance of the Tribunal.

When Dr Ellis reported to his colleagues his failure to assess Andrew Robinson's mental condition, the Tribunal should, we think, have adjourned the hearing. Since Andrew did in fact appear, there would have been little disruption in the proceedings if Dr Ellis had privately examined Andrew there and then. Indeed, it may be that the deficiencies of the hearing, to which we shall have to allude, might have been exposed. Andrew Robinson's ability to manipulate authorities, particularly with his verbal dexterity, would have been less in play when faced with a one-to-one examination. Dr Ellis would also have seen and digested the

information which the nursing staff possessed of Andrew's bizarre,
not to say mad behaviour.

The decision

The Tribunal 'considered the patient's application' and gave four
reasons for discharging Andrew Robinson absolutely:

1. The Tribunal accepts the evidence of Dr Conway that the patient
   is not now suffering from mental illness, nor from any other form
   of mental disorder within the meaning of the Act.

2. The Tribunal is satisfied that the patient has a vulnerable personality, although he is no danger to the public nor himself and he
   does not currently require any treatment.

3. The Tribunal is also satisfied that, should the patient require
   social or medical support in the future he will voluntarily seek
   such help.

4. Accordingly, the Tribunal is satisfied that it is no longer appropriate for the patient to remain liable to be recalled to hospital for
   further treatment.

Ordinarily, an MHRT has to distinguish between the diagnostic
question – whether the patient is still suffering from a mental
disorder – and the policy question, which focuses on the degree of
risk involved in discharging the patient. At the time of Andrew
Robinson's case, it was the commonly-held view that once a patient
was no longer suffering from any mental disorder within the
meaning of the Act, the Tribunal was bound to discharge the
patient from any control. The fact that the patient would need,
psychiatrically or socially, to be under some form of community
supervision would have been irrelevant from the point of view of
Andrew Robinson's Tribunal. Nevertheless, the Tribunal did have
statements from the Home Office and Andrew's supervising officer,
Mr Steven Driscoll, to the effect that they had concern about his
future. The Home Office statement for the consideration of the
MHRT was unequivocal: 'The Home Secretary is satisfied that Mr
Robinson continues to require the guidance and support provided
by his formal supervision in the community and would wish to see
a longer period of stability in the community before he would be
prepared to consider Mr Robinson's absolute discharge. At the

present time the Home Secretary considers that the conditions attached to Mr Robinson's discharge are necessary for his own well being, as well as for the protection of others.'

In his first of three reports to the Home Office on 30 April 1986, Mr Driscoll, after indicating his comparative inability to make contact with Andrew Robinson since becoming responsible for him at the end of 1985, said that Andrew 'has recently displayed some quite paranoid ideas and I do not feel able to recommend that his warrant of conditional discharge should cease at the present time'. The conclusion was not only adverse to the removal of any liability to recall, but it also provided strong contra-indication that Andrew would voluntarily seek 'social or medical support', were he to gain his untrammelled freedom. The Tribunal thought otherwise, even if its conclusion could not have affected its decision, as the law was then thought to be. In his report to the Tribunal on 12 June 1986, without repeating his recommendation, Mr Driscoll seemed to expect that Andrew would be returning to 'some sort of community residence'. In a supplementary report of 8 September 1986, Mr Driscoll merely indicated his efforts to find 'some sort of residential accommodation on discharge'. Mr Driscoll told us that, once the Tribunal had heard that Andrew Robinson was no longer suffering from any mental disorder, any doubts about the wisdom of lifting the restriction order were swept away. That situation could not arise, after June 1989, when the Court of Appeal decided in *R* v. *Merseyside Mental Health Review Tribunal, ex parte K*[3] that a restricted patient who is no longer suffering from a mental disorder remains a 'patient' for the purposes of section 73 (power to discharge restricted patients) until he is discharged absolutely. Even if the patient is no longer suffering from mental illness, the Tribunal is required to direct a conditional discharge unless satisfied that it is inappropriate to recall the patient.

When he referred to 'discharge', Mr Driscoll was contemplating Andrew's discharge from Moorhaven Hospital and not a discharge from the restriction order, even though, strictly speaking, the Tribunal was not, and could not have been dealing with the section 3 admission. Mr Driscoll considered that it was entirely appropriate for a social worker to observe that the patient displayed psychotic features and thought that some consultants at Moorhaven operated in a multi-disciplinary fashion, working closely in teams

[3] [1990] 1 All E.R. 694.

with their professional colleagues, and would listen to the views of colleagues about a patient's mental state. By contrast, Dr Conway represented the old school of psychiatry, compartmentalising the diagnostic question from other aspects of management, the diagnosis being a matter exclusively for the psychiatrist.

Since Dr Ellis, exceptionally in the case of Andrew Robinson, contributed no medical input to the evidence of mental disorder, there remained the sole evidence of Dr Conway, Andrew's RMO for 3 years, as against the accumulated, almost unanimous, psychiatric opinion from 1978 to 1983 in opposition to a diagnosis of personality disorder. Dr Ellis's expertise was limited to an evaluation of Dr Conway's expert evidence. There was no other psychiatric opinion of Andrew's mental condition to hand. Had someone of the calibre of Dr Exworthy prepared a report on the basis of a comprehensive history of psychiatric illness since 1978, such as he did provide to the Crown Court in March 1994, a different result might have evolved.

Why did the Tribunal feel compelled to accept Dr Conway's diagnosis that Andrew Robinson was that of a personality disorder, and not any form of mental disorder, a diagnosis almost uniformly concluded by all Andrew's professional carers? The Tribunal had the uncontroverted opinion of Dr Conway in writing, and confirmed orally by him. Dr Ellis, doubtless, was handicapped in questioning the opinion of someone whose psychiatric standing he respected, since he had been deprived of examining psychiatrically Andrew Robinson himself, as he would have done in the normal course of events. Dr Ellis could, however, have been directed to the nursing and clinical records at Moorhaven which would at least have questioned the state of Andrew Robinson's health. Everything contrived thus to distract the Tribunal from any overview of Andrew's true mental condition. Above all, the Tribunal was greatly disabled by the lack of any historical material about the index offence of 1978 and Dr Udwin's firm diagnosis in 1980 of psychosis requiring long-term supervised medication. Since a tribunal can act only on the material presented to it, we would hope that no MHRT today would be lacking in a complete picture of the patient's psychiatric history. Judge Palmer and his colleagues were presented with the unchallenged evidence of Dr Conway pointing ineluctably to an absolute discharge; they were bound to grant it.

We are finally driven to the conclusion that Dr Conway misled the Tribunal, since his diagnosis of Andrew Robinson's mental condition was palpably faulty. At the very least he should have indicated that his psychiatric opinion was unsupported by any other clinician who had assessed and/or treated Andrew over a number of years. We think that Dr Conway's failure was attributable in part to his long-standing patient-doctor relationship with Andrew.

The mere fact that an RMO has been in a clinical relationship with his/her patient tends to distort the RMO's forensic testimony. The relationship is such that the patient has much to gain by impressing the clinician in a variety of ways. Hence the RMO is in a more powerful and imbalanced role in the relationship than a psychiatrist independently assessing the patient could ever be. The different roles, on the one hand, of assisting and caring for the patient over a long period and, on the other hand, of making a snap analysis and labelling, exacerbated by interviews of short duration and attendant pressures, need to be closely observed and distinguished. All these factors have the potential to distort, even to invalidate the findings by forensic mental health professionals. Dr Conway had, moreover, developed a close, trusting relationship with Andrew. Mr Driscoll described him as 'a very caring and very conscientious consultant who was much loved by his patients'. Dr Ellis also spoke warmly of Dr Conway's professional work – no doubt a factor propelling the Tribunal towards ready acceptance of Dr Conway's evidence. The Tribunal heard, therefore, a very one-sided version of Andrew's psychiatric condition, uncorrected by another, independent opinion or by the other clinicians who had known Andrew in the past.

Dr Conway's role as a 'solo player' – to use Mr Driscoll's words, qualifying the praise for Dr Conway's caring of his patients – was perhaps the decisive feature of his professional work. It blinkered, even blinded him to any modification of his own, palpably suspect opinion of Andrew Robinson's mental health. The habit of disregarding the views of professional colleagues, and a working style which omitted regular multi-disciplinary discussion with others involved in the patient's care, was a serious flaw in his work. And, on this occasion, it fatally led the Tribunal astray.

Part C (2)

Andrew Robinson's Socio-psychiatric History, 1986-1993

X. The Shadow Lengthens: Readmission to and Discharge from Hospital

We have too many high sounding words, and too few actions that correspond with them.*

Within only a few weeks of Andrew Robinson's total freedom from any legal control in September 1986, his father was writing to Dr Conway in desperation about his son's mental state – a refutation of Dr Conway's dubious diagnosis and optimistic prognosis. On 21 October 1986 the Rev. Peter Robinson wrote: 'His [Andrew's] behaviour since he was discharged from hospital has been so *dreadful* that we simply cannot cope any longer. I believe he desperately needs medication. Is there *nothing anyone* can do for him?' The plea for help was repeated in an undated letter to Steven Driscoll, which the latter enclosed in a letter to Dr Conway on 27 October 1986, describing Andrew as 'significantly more paranoid than when we last saw him'. The enclosed letter from the Rev. Peter Robinson read:

> Just to give an example of what we are having to put up with – yesterday afternoon, my wife was listening to 'Woman's Hour' on the radio, when Andrew stormed into the room, smashed the radio to pieces, shouting and swearing at my wife for listening to 'that neo-Nazi terrorist organisation, the BBC'. When I came in from the next room to intervene, he knocked me to the floor and attacked me in a very frightening manner (not for the first time).
> He keeps having 'brain storms' and every day we have continual abuse because we have not sent him abroad.
> I know it will be said nothing can be done without Andrew's consent, but I should be happy for you to show this letter to Dr Conway. I am sure he can have no conception of what we are daily going through – and *have* gone through.

Following the discharge of his compulsory admission by Dr Conway on 17 September and the MHRT's removal on 19 September 1986 of any liability to recall to hospital, Andrew went home

---

* Abigail Adams, letter to John Adams (1774).

with his mother on 25 September 1986. The discharge summary, written by Dr Eadie, SHO to Dr Conway on 2 October 1986, reflected the latter's optimism. It included the following passage:

> During the course of his stay there was nothing to suggest an underlying diagnosis of paranoid schizophrenia and it become more clear that really this was a personality disorder. It also become clear that as a result of his stay in Broadmoor there was no doubt but that he had become psychologically scarred by this experience and that under the circumstances Dr Conway felt that his paranoia was probably justified. He remained well off treatment and during the course of his stay, apart from episodes of frustration which resulted in some verbal disinhibition he never offered any members of staff or patients any violence ...

The importance of the discharge summary should not be underestimated. It is frequently the document upon which a new doctor will base the treatment regime. The gloss that was given to Andrew Robinson's diagnosis, presentation and prognosis was, therefore, highly significant and influential. It stood in stark contrast to every piece of information emanating from the social worker, the nursing staff and Andrew's parents.

The flow of similar information continued. On 9 November 1986 Andrew's GP, Dr Bann, contacted the Social Services Out-of-Hours team, describing a picture of deterioration and requesting a possible admission to Moorhaven Hospital. Dr Conway declined to assess Andrew, as he was now living outside the hospital's catchment area. The following day Dr Moss, a consultant psychiatrist in Torbay District, was contacted. His assessment, as a resulting domiciliary visit on 10 November, was that Andrew had a borderline schizophrenic personality disorder, and that 'it would be best for Andrew to be away from the home situation as quickly as possible'. Arrangements were set in train to secure a supported hostel place for Andrew. Before that became available, on 18 November he was taken to Exminster Hospital by his father and admitted informally under Dr Moss. Dr Moss's statement read:

> During his admission from 18 – 26 November 1986 (Andrew was missing a good deal of the time), he presented as unkempt, aggressive and expressing quite marked paranoid ideas. I felt his mental state was abnormal and unsettled, but not sufficient to detain him, especially as I was trying to establish a relationship with him without appearing immediately unfair and heavy-handed.

In evidence to us he elaborated:

> I think I must have set about trying to establish a therapeutic relationship with Mr Robinson on the basis that he had a personality disorder in which medication might not be the first treatment approach I would use.

When Andrew was discharged on 26 November 1986 a discharge summary was prepared by Dr Cullen, SHO to Dr Moss. This discharge summary, in addition to several factual errors, stated Andrew's diagnosis as personality disorder.

On 29 November 1986 Andrew was readmitted – his first admission to EMC – under the care of Dr Moss on a section 4 of the Mental Health Act 1983 (an emergency admission for assessment). The reasons given for this admission were:

1. Has assaulted his parents
2. Believes village woman has cast spell ('parapsychologist') and is using occult power to control his mind and block his thoughts.
3. Has declared his intention to kill this women to rid himself of her influence.

On 1 December 1986 the emergency admission was converted, first to a section 2 order (for assessment) and on 23 December to a section 3 order (for treatment). When Dr Moss wrote his report to the MHRT on 10 December 1986, he concluded: 'In my view, he has now shown clearly that his earlier tendency to schizophrenia is still very much a reality to be reckoned with, and he needs treatment in hospital until he can be trusted to cope appropriately outside hospital, and to take medication as necessary.'

In his written statement to the Inquiry, confirmed in oral evidence, Dr Moss declared: 'My diagnosis has remained one of paranoid schizophrenia.'

Consistent with the diagnosis of paranoid schizophrenia, Andrew was put on antipsychotic drugs which had a marked beneficial effect. Andrew regularly protested about having to take medication, and made frequent attempts to have it reduced or altered. Each reduction, however, produced a deterioration in his mental state. By March 1987 he had settled, to the extent that a community placement was considered appropriate for him, and he was referred on 25 March 1987 to Cypress rehabilitation hostel. He was assessed on 9 April 1987, the record of that assessment including the following: 'When asked what his plans were, he was quite clear

– to live independently of any agency connected with mental health, and to come off medication, which he claims is controlling constructive thought.' Later in the same report: 'We asked him what brought him to the EMC. He became vague, talked of witchcráft and Black Magic and demonstrated no insight whatsoever into his condition.'

Andrew was offered a placement at Cypress which was taken up on 22 April 1987. He was regarded as being on leave of absence from EMC, and his section 3 remained in place until it lapsed on 22 June 1987. The purpose of this assessment was to make a judgment about the necessity of continuing the section. It was felt that in the light of his improvement the continuation of the section was not justified. The dilemma facing Dr Moss was spelled out in a letter that he wrote to Andrew's father on 8 May 1987:

> Like yourself, I am concerned with his threats not to continue with the medication once there is no compulsion for him to do so. The whole situation is a very difficult one, because while it is technically possible to detain him in hospital accommodation for a longer period of time, I suspect that this might detract from Andrew's progress rather than aiding it therapeutically.
>
> In my view, much the best policy is to continue to try to persuade Andrew through advice and personal experience that life is actually more equable when he is taking the medication. In the event this may mean more periods in hospital under detention until the penny drops.

Although there was widespread recognition that Andrew was likely to refuse medication, when no longer compelled to comply with the Mental Health Act, this was not a situation that had previously occurred. When in the past Andrew discontinued medication, it had been at the direction of his RMO. It was just possible that, as an informal patient, he would comply with prescribed treatment. In the event this proved not to be the case. Three days after the compulsory admission lapsed, he left Cypress and moved to Exeter, all medication discontinued. Dr Moss wrote to a consultant psychiatrist in Exeter who agreed to take over Andrew's care, but was unable to make contact with him. Andrew's condition deteriorated and he was readmitted to EMC for the second time on 18 December 1987 under Dr Orr, for assessment. By 18 February 1988 he had been discharged. Throughout the admission there was a lack of clarity about medical responsibility. Dr Orr referred to himself as the 'nominal RMO' and relied on his Senior Registrar, Dr Parke, to be 'virtually responsible for the clinical care'. Dr Orr acknowledged to us that it is not right to refer to an RMO as being only 'nominally' responsible for the patient. The responsibility is not delegable. There were certain troubling aspects relating to this period of care. Andrew had been admitted with delusional ideas about witchcraft and being influenced by a woman neighbour. He had written to the Bishop requesting exorcism, and on 22 December 1987 there was a nursing note: 'Visit by the Rev. Martin Shaw, Bishop's Envoy, to deal with exorcism/paranormal. Did not see Andrew. Saw Dr Parke who said he would prefer to see Andrew when he was a little better.' When we asked about his view of an exorcist attending a patient with pathological beliefs about possession, telepathy and witchcraft while in hospital, Dr Orr commented: 'I can remember two or three episodes where patients, usually long-term patients with religious delusions and hallucinations, are very distressed by what they feel to be possession by the devil and we have organised exorcism. It usually does not have much effect.' Such a stance appears to us to be collusive and potentially very damaging.

On 29 December Andrew absented himself from EMC without leave of his RMO. An entry in the medical notes stated: 'Dr Orr informed – feels Andrew is a risk to women in Stoke Fleming and ex-girlfriend in Exeter – Police informed.'

Andrew was returned to EMC by the police on 31 December. On 13 January he was interviewed by Dr Parke with respect to a section 3 application. The record showed: 'Admits to being influenced by this woman although less so. Talks of sexual relations with this woman although she will probably call it "Rape".' Dr Parke's opinion was that Andrew 'will accept medical advise [sic] on staying as in-patient for up to six weeks or thereabouts and will also take medication'. Section 3 was not felt to be required. The view taken by Dr Parke on medication appears to be somewhat optimistic when a comparison is made between what is prescribed at this period and what was actually administered. Difficulty over medication is further noted in the entry following the ward round on 19 January 1988: 'Accepting medication after some argument' and following the clinical review on 16 February 1988, the nursing note read: 'Sulpiride stopped as he probably won't take it when he is discharged.'

The overall impression, conveyed by the medical and nursing notes, the written statements and the oral evidence relating to this period of Andrew's care is that there was a sad lack of clear and

consistent planning for Andrew's immediate treatment in hospital
and for his longer-term treatment in the community. There was a
general sense of him posing a risk to two women in the community,
but little evidence of thorough risk-assessment and risk-management in relation to this threat.

Following his discharge, Andrew went to a bed and breakfast in
Paignton. He received no further medication until he was readmitted informally, again under Dr Orr, on 9 May 1988. On 10 May
Andrew again went absent without leave and did not return until
13 May when he was located in his Paignton flat and was persuaded
by the police to return to EMC. Andrew remained as an informal
patient, although there were frequent references in the nursing
and medical notes about 'sectioning' him if he tried to leave or
refused medication. From the notes that do exist, and there would
appear to be a section of the medical notes at least that are missing,
Andrew continued to present marked psychotic features. On 22
May 1988 there was reference to his continuing preoccupation with
his nose, and the same entry continued: 'Andrew feels that the only
way to fight the system is to "kill someone" and then people might
respect him a bit more.' The entry for the following day continued:
'Seen by Dr Parke today who feels that Andrew is psychotic (extremely) and very unwell at the moment. If Andrew wishes to leave
he is to be sectioned under the MHA.' In his evidence to us Dr Orr
conceded: 'I did feel it rather curious, yes, that here they are saying
that he was really quite disturbed and then three or four weeks
later he is fit for discharge.'

Despite the experience from the previous discharge from EMC,
and Andrew's rapid default in medication accompanied by swift
deterioration in his mental health, there was once again a lack of
evidence of clear and consistent planning around Andrew's immediate care, and around longer-term care in the community. Andrew
was permitted to take his own discharge on 24 June 1988, returning
to a bed and breakfast in Paignton. His medical care was transferred to Dr Moss, who had catchment-area responsibility for that
patch. There was no clarity about the arrangements that had been
made for community follow-up, particularly relating to the administration of depot medication. For a low-risk client, this would be
poor practice. For a high-risk client like Andrew an outpatient
appointment was necessary. This was done and Dr Moss saw
Andrew on 20 July 1988, four weeks after Andrew had left EMC.
In a letter to Andrew's GP Dr Moss wrote: 'He told me that he has

avoided medication since he left hospital.' He continued: 'He feels that he suffers from a paranormal experience which he puts down to demon possession ... I doubt whether he will be able to avoid further admissions to hospital.'

On 2 August 1988 Jackie Wright, CPN, went to assess Andrew at the Paignton bed and breakfast, at the request of her manager, Iain Tulley. It was intended that Mrs Wright should take over the role of key worker. In her written statement to the Inquiry, Mrs Wright stated:

> Having read the records I was unhappy about this proposal in principle, partly because of the incident in 1978 with the shotgun and partly because of the apparent obsession with Mrs A. I was even more unhappy after I had met Mr Robinson and I declined to become his key worker because:
>
> 1. He did not want any contact with the psychiatric services, because (he said) they represented hospitals and medication, and because they did not understand him, and
>
> 2. I had found him very intimidating, to an extent which I have never experienced with any other patient, before or since.

Les Grainger was appointed as Andrew's key worker. Between August and November 1988 there was a noticeable deterioration. On 14 October 1988 Mrs Robinson phoned Jackie Wright expressing great concern about Andrew. Mrs Robinson reported to Jackie Wright that Andrew had said 'he was trapped under this elderly woman's powers and found it hard to escape ... she (Mrs Robinson) said Andrew was dangerous and needed admission to hospital'. Mrs Wright and Mr Grainger visited Andrew, but no further action was taken. On 21 October Andrew's landlady found an air pistol in his room. Iain Tulley was contacted and, in turn, informed Dr Moss. Mr Tulley took the gun to the local police and carried out an assessment on Andrew. Mr Tulley's account in the notes stated:

> Andrew was quite composed and answered questions quite appropriately. He said, when asked about the gun, 'it made me look macho', at which point he blushed ... We left Andrew feeling that there was little that could or in fact needed done.

Mr Tulley told us that after making his assessment he reported back to Dr Moss. He also stated that he had been unaware at the

time that Andrew's index offence had involved the discharging of
a firearm, although he had been aware that there had been a threat
with a shotgun.

On 3 November 1988 Andrew's father wrote to Dr Moss: 'He is
again very unwell. It is 5 months since he was last in hospital and
received any medication, and, as usual he is starting again to
hallucinate badly, saying he is possessed by Mrs A. ... I feel the
time has come when he must receive medication again, compulsorily if necessary.' On 11 November 1988 Andrew was admitted
to EMC under section 2. This was his fourth admission within 2
years. The admission note read:

> Admitted now from Torquay police station under section 2 of M.H.A
> 1983. Has been writing threatening letters to a particular lady in
> Stoke Gabriel. This problem has continued apparently over the last
> 3 years. Arrested following further letters. Fixed paranoid delusion
> about this woman ... No apparent reason for this:

> 'I advised her about her soul'
> 'It was a political move'
> 'She fell in love with me'
> 'It was intended to get rid of her for good – she'll burn' ...

The problems produced by inadequate or distorted communication
around key facts is revealed later on in the same entry. Although
it was stated that Andrew was 'well known to the unit', under the
heading, 'previous psychiatric history', there appeared the comment: 'Apparently threatened someone with a gun and admitted to
Broadmoor "section 65"?'

On 14 November 1988 Iain Tulley wrote to Dr Moss, commenting
on the extreme difficulty that he and his team had had in maintaining any 'meaningful contact' with Andrew in the community.
He continued:

> Can I suggest that during his stay in hospital this time, we look
> toward a guardianship order prior to his discharge, His landlady is
> in close contact with the Cypress team and is prepared to have him
> back. With guardianship we maybe able to exercise some sort of
> control over his situation.

There is an entry in the EMC notes of the same day:

> Phone call from Iain Tulley re Andrew. Would like a guardianship

order to be strongly considered to keep some tabs on Andrew in the community. Feels he is a danger left unsupervised.

On 8 December 1988 Dr Moss reviewed the case:

In general I think he is better than on admission, or on his last discharge from our care in hospital. But in view of the public alarm about him, I feel we have to make sure of him by keeping him here on section 3 with a view either to guardianship and maintenance medication, or a further trial off medication (which I don't believe he is yet ready for).

Seven days later Andrew was regraded to section 3.

During this period Mrs A. was becoming so distressed with Andrew's continuing harassment that she instructed a local solicitor to act for her. He wrote on several occasions to Dr Moss and finally met with him on 27 January 1989. This was recorded as a 'most helpful meeting'. We were told: 'At that meeting he [Dr Moss] had modified his opinion from one of guarded scepticism to one where he now said he agreed, he was now convinced there was a serious problem.' The solicitor, Mr Hansell, further confirmed that in November 1989, when Andrew was due to be discharged, Dr Moss contacted him to inform him of the discharge arrangements.

In his evidence to us, Mr Hansell expressed the following view which we regard as commendable. We, therefore, record it in full:

I think the first problem is actually finding out the reality of the situation. We knew of certain stories about what had happened to him in the past. I had no way of verifying those. I wrote to Broadmoor Hospital and asked them and got the brush-off. As you can see Dr Moss gave me an indication there were matters of confidentiality that I couldn't be told, so I felt as Mrs A.'s adviser I wasn't being told everything. Now it could be there ware very good reasons for not telling me anything. I don't know. That is outside my brief. However, I feel that, looked at from Mrs A.'s point of view, it might have been some direct communication. I think in the first place somebody in authority should have gone to see her, spoken to her directly, as I would interviewing a witness. The first thing you want to know is what is the credibility of the person. I am taking statements from people every day of the week and some of them one takes slightly tongue in cheek, knowing the person is probably unreliable and is making half of it up. Other people you take a statement from you get a feeling there is truth in it and you can assess that person.

I would like to think that in the future if anything like this happened, whoever feels concerned should at least have the courtesy of a visit. I know there are constraints on finance and facilities, but it might be that a lot of those concerns can be set at rest, especially in the world of mental health, which is fairly complicated. Even I, as a lawyer, would struggle to understand in parts. So a greater degree of communication, some way of expressing concern without having to rush off to solicitors, might be a help.

Although he did not meet Mrs A., Dr Moss did take steps to gather information about Andrew's behaviour in relation to her by writing to Andrew's GP and to the local police. In response to the request for information and opinion Dr Lockerbie, the GP, wrote back on 4 January 1989: 'I am of the belief, and so is Dr Orr, that Andrew is quite capable of carrying out his threat of killing or sexually assaulting Mrs A.' As the evidence was gathered, Dr Moss became increasingly concerned for Mrs A.'s safety. In the EMC notes of 13 December 1988 Dr Moss wrote: 'We have now seen a letter he has written to Mrs A., almost certainly since admission. It indicates thought patterns far more sinister than he is revealing on the surface. ... This means that we must continue to keep him under careful supervision.'

During the period from November 1986 to February 1989 Andrew had four separate admissions to EMC. Each one was marked by a disturbed and psychotic presentation, preceded by a medication-free period. The first and third admissions were informal, and from the first three Andrew effectively discharged himself. A clear pattern had become established. Without compulsory powers Andrew would default on any treatment programme. If he was not taking his medication, Andrew's mental state would progressively worsen.

XI. Respite and Warning: The Butler Clinic, February – August 1989

Making mental connections is a most crucial learning tool, the essence of human intelligence to forge links; to go beyond the given; to see patterns, relationship, context.*

On 1 February 1989 Dr Moss, now of the view that Andrew Robinson required greater security than EMC could offer, wrote to Dr Martin Donovan, the Principal Consultant Psychiatrist at the local Regional Secure Unit, the Butler Clinic, in Dawlish, South Devon, asking for an assessment of Andrew Robinson with a view to his transfer there. Dr Moss wrote in his statement to the Inquiry: 'During this admission I took active steps to establish the degree of threat posed to Mrs A. I started out trying to be fair to Mr Robinson's legitimate interests, but it became quite clear that he was again blaming Mrs A. for his problems to the extent that she was a possible target of his paranoid behaviour. My ward staff then made me aware that I too was becoming a target, and at this point I requested his admission to the Butler Clinic so greater security could be exercised.'

On 10 February 1989 Dr Patrick Gallwey, consultant forensic psychiatrist working at the Butler Clinic, came to assess Andrew Robinson. He found that Andrew had no insight into his mental illness, aggression or dangerousness, and thought that Andrew was very obviously playing down his aggressiveness and dangerousness. Dr Gallwey agreed to admit Andrew to the Butler Clinic to assess his dangerousness, and to see whether his delusional system could be modified. Andrew Robinson was transferred to the Butler Clinic three days later and stayed there for just under six months.

On admission he was noted to be experiencing frank delusional ideas, particularly delusions of passivity and control by Mrs A. After a brief period off medication, which followed the discovery of modestly abnormal liver function tests (a frequent untoward response to chlorpromazine), he was treated with chlorpromazine

* Marilyn Ferguson, *The Aquarian Conspiracy* (1980).

800 mg a day, reducing over a period of 2 to 3 weeks to 200 mg a day. He remained floridly psychotic for some weeks, but gradually began to improve. His delusional ideas gradually abated, although he remained odd and preoccupied throughout his stay. His behaviour towards women caused considerable anxiety, and the content of his writing was bizarrely sadistic. On 8 April 1989 a staff nurse found a note typed by Andrew Robinson which described a homicidal plan of truly gruesome detail, set out with a clarity of thought which makes the reading of it the more chilling. We reproduce it here in exactly the form in which it was uncovered.

```
I had to think up a torture for Mrs ████.I thought I should tie
her up th en approach her with a power driven chain saw and cut off her
fungersxixxxx of one hand. I would f ed her them to keep her alive.
Then I wou d saw off her hand for her next meal.I would go on up the
arm sawing off slices to :eep her alive for a week.I would start on nhe
her other aarm rthen her legs.I would then use her as a dart board
and see her hob bl ng about on her stumps to try and avoid the
darts. I wou d aim for plafes like the eye.I would then hang her up
from the celing by her hair giving her jus t enough to eat to stay
alive and keep her t ere f or ten or twenty years, however long it
took for her to die.

        should someone ask, do yoy be i eve in the paranormal would be
        asking as basic a question as,  do you believe in television?.
```

When Dr Gallwey was asked at the Inquiry about the note he said that all the staff were alarmed by the document, as they were about 'others comparable to that'. Dr Gallwey said that it was always 'very, very worrying when you get this strongly sadistic element in florid psychosis', adding that the markedly sadistic and homicidal ideation had been first observed in Andrew really in late 1986. Dr Moss, who had never seen the typed note before 25 July 1994 at the oral hearing of the Inquiry, said that it would have had a considerable impact on him, adding that he too would have been alarmed by the homicidal, sadistic ideation exhibited by Andrew Robinson. And Dr McLaren, when shown the document at the Inquiry, likewise expressed the view that he could not have failed to be affected in the way he would have viewed Andrew Robinson in June 1993.

On 5 June 1989, when Andrew Robinson was thought to be improving in terms of his psychotic experiences, the clinical notes recorded:

> *Nurses*: overfamiliar with female staff (esp. S.), asking to marry and asking what they do when they orgasm etc., told off, but persists. Even said wanted to tie up nurse and abuse her. Invasive, erotically unwelcome; repeating [history] of overdependence which has at times led to threats with gun; female nurses *shouldn't* be alone with him. Encourage female nurses to disengage from him, and *not* to read his autobiographical book (some of which is 'disgusting').
> *Dr G*: nurses must ensure male staff are with S. when patient is around.
> For community parole with 2 escorts.

That this specialist clinic noted that female nurses should not be alone with Andrew Robinson may be important. We do not know whether the guidance for nurses was followed consistently while he was at the Butler Clinic, but it shows a degree of alarm about the possible threat he represented to female staff. It is perhaps as well to remember, however, that Andrew Robinson was in the less secure part of the clinic by June, and was granted escorted leave in the community, so presumably staff at the clinic cannot have felt that he was a serious risk to women in general.

His preoccupation with one nurse, and the precautions taken, were reported in the discharge summary, prepared by Dr Gallwey's clinical assistant, Dr Umar, and sent to EMC after his transfer back there. There is, however, no mention in the transfer note that accompanied Andrew Robinson back to EMC of the decision not to allow female nurses to be alone with him. If anything, Dr Umar's discharge summary is rather reassuring, since it concluded:

> During his stay here he did not show any physical aggression towards staff or fellow patients. He maintained his improvement. The patient was discharged in a satisfactory and much improved mental state ...

Dr Moss visited Andrew Robinson at the Butler Clinic twice, once on 11 May 1989 to renew his detention under section 3, and again on 20 July to discuss his progress and possible transfer back to EMC. There is no record in the clinical notes that Andrew

Robinson's attitude to female staff was discussed at the case
conference on 20 July. Certainly, Dr Moss does not recall that it
was, and in all likelihood the subject was not raised. Dr Moss did
not recall Dr Gallwey being present at the case conference on 20
July and, in fact, did not think he had ever attended a case
conference on a patient at the Butler Clinic when Dr Gallwey had
been present, because most of Dr Moss's patients had been cared
for by Dr Donovan. It seems likely, bearing in mind Dr Gallwey's
memorable style, and the fact that his presence is not noted in the
clinical notes, that he was not present at this case conference and
did not, therefore, have an opportunity to convey to Dr Moss his
anxieties about Andrew Robinson's potential risk to women. Dr
Moss would surely have remembered such an event.

Dr Gallwey in his evidence to us was quite clear that at the case
conference he would have expected nurses to have raised the issue
with Dr Moss and any accompanying members of the team from
EMC. When asked by Mr Thorold: 'Is it in your view inconceivable,
therefore, that at the meeting with Dr Moss this would not have
been discussed orally, that nurses would have actually raised this
issue about that note?' he replied:

> Yes, absolutely. From early on we realised that he was very over-
> aroused by female staff. I had a confrontation with him over it and
> he became very angry with me because earlier on in his stay when
> he was more psychotic he was in fact assaulting nurses actually.

> Q. Female only?

> Female nurses, yes, and he, of course, said he would kill me and so
> forth. You have to stress, of course, that in our unit that isn't a very
> unusual occurrence. One constantly, well not constantly, but often,
> has death threats from patients, and so do the nurses, and also one
> has alarmingly sadistic material coming. I am not saying that he
> stands out ...

The Chairman then interrupted: 'He was not exceptional?' to which
Dr Gallwey replied:

> ... alone or exceptional. He is not every-day, by any means, but he is
> certainly not an exception in that way. Where I think I was very
> reassured, and I think Dr Moss was at that time, was in his very
> good and clear response to the neuroleptics and also, I think, to our
> regime ...

So we conclude that while Dr Gallwey would, if he had been present, have conveyed the risk he perceived Andrew Robinson to be to female staff to Dr Moss at the case conference, he was not in fact present that day, and Dr Moss would have agreed to his transfer back to EMC in the knowledge of Andrew Robinson's good response to medication, but with no special anxieties about Andrew Robinson's attitude to female staff. He would have been further reassured by Dr Umar's discharge summary, albeit with some knowledge from the summary that Andrew Robinson had exhibited worrying behaviour towards a nurse at some point during the admission. Andrew Robinson had been on successful escorted leave from the Butler Clinic, and Dr Moss must have felt quite satisfied that the time had come for the general psychiatric service to resume its responsibility for Andrew Robinson's care.

It is difficult to judge whether Dr Moss would have felt differently, had he read the clinical notes in full personally, or if the notes had been transferred with Andrew Robinson when he moved to EMC, instead of the discharge summary that was supplied. It seems possible that, if EMC nurses had had access to the full nursing records made by their colleagues at the Butler Clinic, their plan for him might have been modified in the light of their greater knowledge. At present it is not the practice for RSU or Special Hospital notes to transfer to the patient's next 'port of call', and it would be unusual for a visiting consultant to read through all the notes; he would place his faith in the opinions of professionals expressed directly at the case conference.

Just as it would be unnecessary in a medical discharge note to state that an insulin-dependent diabetic would require insulin for the rest of his life, so it would be unnecessary for Dr Umar to remark on Andrew Robinson's future need for continued neuroleptic medication in the light of the diagnosis of schizophrenia. The dose of clopixol decanoate (depot neuroleptic) on discharge is recorded as 300 mg intramuscularly every two weeks, with orphenadrine 50 mg daily for extra-pyramidal side effects. Dr Gallwey concurred with the view put to him that, in order to prevent Andrew Robinson becoming psychotic once more, it was essential to keep him on long-term medication, but cautioned, in response to Mr Thorold's further question: 'Would it therefore have been your view that if he ever stopped taking medication that those in touch with him would have to intervene very speedily?'

Well, obviously only if they could. It would mean that you would have to be especially watchful, and the first signs of the psychosis re-emerging then you would need to take charge of him. You can't admit somebody who won't be admitted unless they are showing sufficient evidence that they require attention. Obviously it is a *sine qua non* of intervention that the person either agrees or that they have a mental disorder of a kind that enables you to invoke the Mental Health Act, so clearly what he required was very long-term monitoring, and action as necessary.

The Chairman then asked: 'And persistent medication?'

And to keep him on the medication and obviously only take it off very gradually and then reinstate it if there was any sign of a recurrence. You can't keep somebody on medicine forever if they are all right. You have got to reduce it, and people, of course, as you will know, Sir Louis, and everyone here with any knowledge of mental illness will know, that you can't say that people do not get better. You can't, as it were, presume that somebody is going to do something. It is one of the great dilemmas of psychiatry. A lot of it is taking action on presumption. People lose their freedom not because of what they have done but because one is frightened of what they might do. That is, I think, a cause of some concern amongst libertarians who feel that gives psychiatrists a power that they can misuse. So I think we are all very, very keen not to take premature action. Having said that, however, this man obviously fell into a category of patient one would want to be jolly alert about.

Dr Gallwey neatly sums up in these paragraphs the dilemmas that faced Dr Moss and other consultants who treated Andrew Robinson in the years after his transfer back from the Butler Clinic to EMC.

It is worth noting one other point of interest in the Butler Clinic notes. A nurse recorded on 26 June that Andrew Robinson had said his father had told him Mrs A. was dead. In fact, his father did not impart this piece of information. But whatever the source, whether it was from within Andrew Robinson's own psyche or from an unknown external source, he may, in consequence, have been relieved of part of his mental burden.

XII. The Shadow Shortens:
Guardianship, 1989-1992

The Christian ideal has not been tried and found wanting. It has
been found difficult; and left untried.*

On Andrew Robinson's return from the Butler Clinic to EMC on 1
August 1989, Dr Moss noted that his patient was 'considerably
improved'. In his statement to us Dr Moss reported that he had had
some anxieties about the lack of appropriate activities for Mr
Robinson in EMC. At the Butler Clinic, he had been occupied with
educational sessions; no such comparable facilities were available
at EMC. But, overall, Dr Moss was content that his patient should
return. On 4 August he reviewed Andrew's progress and made a
brief, but clinically comprehensive note of action to be taken by
members of the clinical team. The care plan was as follows.

First, to 'negotiate' with Cypress hostel for a place for Andrew
in the near future; secondly, to look into possible educational
courses which he might follow, this to be discussed with the local
Disablement Resettlement Officer (DRO) and careers service;
thirdly, and importantly, to 'prepare for Guardianship'; and fourthly, to ask Dr Gillespie, a consultant colleague with a special
interest in psychopharmacology, to review Andrew's drug regime
and to consider whether any alternative anti-psychotic might reduce his akathisia and drug-related movement disorder.

Guardianship

Dr Moss's decision to consider a Guardianship Order as a framework to provide appropriate care in the community was both
unusual and commendable. No one could recall the making of a
Guardianship Order in South Devon for a severely mentally disordered patient. Dr Moss wrote at the time: 'I think a guardianship
order may well be a suitable way to negotiate a reasonably early

* G.K. Chesterton, 'What's wrong with the World' from *The Unfinished Temple*
(1910).

discharge from hospital.' The word 'negotiate' is the key word, on which the success of the strategy depended.

Three days after his return to EMC, Andrew Robinson had applied to a MHRT for a discharge. Dr Moss was by no means confident that the Tribunal would reject the application. The nursing notes record that Dr Moss 'feels that Andrew may well be successful as actual threatening behaviour is "history" rather than current ...', and in his evidence to us he noted: 'I felt obliged to make use of the only provision in the Mental Health Act 1983 which comes anywhere near to what I considered Mr Robinson needed, namely Guardianship.' In the event, the Tribunal rejected Andrew's appeal against his section 3 admission. The Guardianship Order was implemented, after much negotiation with officers of Devon Social Services, in November 1989 on his discharge from hospital. The order was in force until it was removed in July 1992.

The Guardianship Order proved to be successful in providing an appropriate framework for Andrew Robinson's care. It is worth considering in some detail how and why it worked, since it has so far been under-used, and official encouragement for its wider application is on the agenda for mental health policy-making. (The role of Guardianship will be considered in greater depth in Chapter XXI.)

In England and Wales, there are approximately 200 Guardianship Orders implemented each year[1] and the majority are used to provide care for people with learning disabilities or older people with dementia. Section 8 of the Mental Health Act 1983 confers on the guardian:

(a) the power to require the patient to reside at a place specified by the authority or person named as guardian

(b) the power to require the patient to attend at places and times so specified for the purpose of medical treatment, occupation, education or training although, unlike its statutory predecessor (the 1959 Act), it contained no power to convey; and

(c) the power to require access to the patient to be given at any place where the patient is residing, to any registered medical practitioner, approved social worker or other person so specified.

Guardianship does not, however, allow for treatment, such as

[1] Department of Health Annual Statistical Returns. Guardianship Orders under Section 7 and Section 37 of the Mental Health Act 1983.

depot medication, to be given without consent, a reason cited frequently for its non-use in patients with mental illness. Dr Moss stressed that in Andrew Robinson's case everyone involved in the decision was well aware of the limitations of the order.

> I therefore took the view that having set an explicit care plan/'contract', default was defined and could be acted upon by the use of readmission under Section 2, if that became necessary. I note that the contractual agreement did not spell out my insistence that Mr Robinson continue to receive his injections, presumably because I was not an immediate party to the agreement, though I supervised it closely.

The contractual arrangement, which Dr Moss felt was crucial to the success of the order, was made between Andrew Robinson, Carol Moore, his landlady in Paignton, medical and nursing staff at EMC, and staff at Cypress Hostel, where Andrew would be attending for meals at weekends. The contract is remarkably detailed in setting out Andrew's domestic and personal responsibilities, his attendance at the Britannia Centre, his agreement to be seen every week by Les Grainger, his CPN, and a number of other conditions, including 'not to be in possession of any offensive weapons' and not to visit Stoke Fleming, Mrs A.'s home village. Carol Moore's and Les Grainger's responsibilities are also spelled out, the latter having the key task of liaising with Dr Moss.

Andrew Robinson was undoubtedly content, if unenthusiastic about complying with the plan. Shortly after discharge, Dr Moss reviewed him at the community team base, Culverhay in Paignton, and noted: '... amazingly content with himself (95% on a scale towards his ideal!). Accepting the contract.'

Andrew accepted depot medication injections, a fairly modest dose of Clopixol 300 mg, given every three weeks by Les Grainger. This continued until the end of 1991. We are confident that Andrew understood the terms of his Guardianship Order because he told us so when we interviewed him at Broadmoor on 30 June 1994. He told us that he had written to the Mental Health Act Commission to check his position with regard to his consent to medication. We confirmed that on 1 July 1991 he wrote to the Commission to clarify whether or not he had to accept treatment, expressing his view that the Clopixol was harmful to him and of no benefit. He received a reply from the Commission dated 15 July 1991, drafted by a Commission member, Mr Richard Lingham, which set out very clearly that the order did not empower medical treatment. We conclude that he was aware of the terms of the Guardianship Order from the outset.

Why then did Andrew Robinson accept medication during the period of the Guardianship Order? The answer undoubtedly lies in the relationship which he had with members of the team who were responsible for his care and his understanding of the supervisory control they exerted over aspects of his life under the Order. He told us when we saw him that he did not want to upset them by refusing to cooperate. If this is a coercive mechanism for ensuring that a patient may be treated in the community, then it is coercion of a very positive kind and surely one of the major benefits conferred by the Order.

Robert Steer, the social worker member of the team who supervised the Order on behalf of the guardian, Devon Social Services, gave us his view of the order: 'I would say that the reason it was successful was because the guardianship allowed the staff to build a relationship for the first time.' The key contact was Les Grainger, who visited Andrew every week, until the role of key worker was assumed in August 1991 by State Enrolled Nurse John Camus. He continued to play a crucially supportive role in the events of Andrew Robinson's life right up to the fatal event of 1 September 1993. John Camus had known Andrew previously when he was employed at Exminster Hospital in the patients' recreation centre in 1986, and later their paths had crossed again, quite by chance in 1987 when Mr Camus was running the Britannia Day Centre which Andrew was attending. Mr Camus was sympathetic to Andrew's plight and probably formed as good a relationship with him as was conceivably possible. Mr Camus's warm, avuncular approach was undoubtedly a major factor in Andrew's trust in the team during the year following. When asked if he would identify the reason for the success of the Guardianship Order as being a consequence of his good rapport with Andrew, Mr Camus replied: 'Partly that and partly that Andrew was always aiming to be free from – his long term aim was to be free from the psychiatric service, so he would play ball, he would cooperate.' The appropriate word to use in this context might be 'engagement' – Andrew Robinson was sufficiently 'engaged' with John Camus and other team members to allow them effectively to discharge their responsibilities.

From Andrew's parents' point of view, the Guardianship Order appeared to work fairly well. The Rev. Peter Robinson wrote to Devon Social Services just after the order was made:

> We are pleased that a Guardianship Order has been placed on Andrew and trust it will be renewed as long as necessary. It would be unbearable to go back to the situation we faced for years, with Andrew continuously going on and off medication, and with the inevitable relapse that followed each time he refused to accept medication voluntarily.

When asked by Mr Thorold if he had any observations about why compliance with medication was achievable under an order that didn't in fact have legal teeth, Mr Robinson replied: 'I can't. I think he just felt he wanted to remain on good terms with his social workers, and for that reason he thought it better to comply. However, as you say, it had no teeth, really.'

It would be wrong to imply that Andrew's progress under the Order was all plain sailing. His initial high spirits on discharge from hospital in November 1989 were not sustained. His landlady, Carol Moore, became increasingly concerned about his poor self-care, the squalid state of his room and his eccentric behaviour – he would come up behind her and just stand there. He shouted and banged objects around his room in a puzzling way. It is interesting to note that Carol Moore never felt in the least threatened by him, even in 1988 (before Guardianship was in place) when a gun and cartridges were found in his room: 'At no time did I feel Mr Robinson to be a real threat to either myself or my family'; and she confirmed this again at the Inquiry, although she admitted she felt Andrew was trying at times to intimidate her.

The episode of self-harm, April 1992

By February 1990, however, Les Grainger noted that Carol Moore felt Andrew Robinson's mental state was deteriorating. Reports of banging and shouting and neglect of his domestic responsibilities continued throughout February and March. Dr Moss at one point considered whether a section 2 admission was warranted. Andrew was noted to be complying with medication and attending the Britannia Centre regularly, but adhering to little else in the contract. He was actively psychotic at this time; he told Robert Steer at the end of January: 'Roger Moss has stolen my soul.' While there was some improvement, noted by Dr Moss on 4 April, he was

admitted to the Intensive Care Unit at Torbay General Hospital
after taking a large, potentially lethal quantity (70) of orphenadrine tablets and was subsequently admitted to EMC on 11
April, having been transferred during the night because of the
inability of the ITU staff to cope with his extreme restlessness and
lack of cooperation. He was still suffering the toxic confusional
effects of the overdose on transfer, and remained acutely confused
for some days. The reasons for his taking the overdose are not clear;
but he admitted that he had been making a serious attempt to end
his life, but was also making a 'cry for help' in the face of perceived
persecution by the 'police and media'.

Moving house and Guardianship reviewed

Andrew Robinson was unable to return to his lodgings at Mrs
Moore's house after the admission in April 1990, and he was
unwilling to consider a placement at Cypress again. After much
effort, a place was found at St Andrew's Lodge, an independent
sector hostel in Paignton. He continued his medication and attendance at the Britannia Centre, but remained deluded and a constant source of worry to his parents, who wrote frequently
throughout the autumn of 1990 to Dr Moss to express their concern
about Andrew's mental state, especially when he became obsessed
once more with a woman, Miss S., about whom he was writing
sadistic notes.

Andrew Robinson's fragile condition compelled the renewal of
the Guardianship Order. It was duly renewed in December 1991,
and his application to the MHRT to be discharged from the Order
was refused on 22 April 1991. Dr Moss's report to the Tribunal,
dated 18 March 1991, concludes:

> No significant improvement in Andrew Robinson's condition has
> been reported to me since I last saw him. I am well aware that he
> feels that his past history of contact with psychiatric services and
> detention under the Mental Health Act acts as a major handicap for
> him. Nevertheless, he persistently fails to take advantage of the
> opportunity he has to demonstrate that he can order his life reliably,
> without threat to others, and he does very little to secure any trust
> that he could now do better than he has done in the past when he
> has lived on his own.
>   I believe that since he left Broadmoor Hospital every effort has
> been made to give him opportunities to prove himself in the commu-
> nity, as well as through further long periods of treatment in hospital.

He has responded to this help only up to the point I have described above. I feel that the only realistic alternative to his present placement is for him to be detained in a more hospital-like environment, and neither he nor we would wish this for him if that can possibly be avoided. I therefore consider that it is vital that the Guardianship Order is continued until he can demonstrate over a period of time that he can take much more responsibility for himself. Because his basic attitudes are only at best partially resolved, I believe that, without regular supervision and medication, there must remain a significant risk to the safety of members of the public.

A period of relative stability followed the rejection of Andrew's appeal. He moved in August 1991 from St Andrew's Lodge to a group home, and for the next six months was judged by Robert Steer, John Camus, who was now his key worker, and Dr Moss to be gradually improving. The dose of Clopixol was reduced slightly in January 1992; such was Andrew's apparent cooperation that Dr Moss ruminated about the possibility of his transferring in the future to a relatively new, but potent anti-psychotic, Clozapine, which since it can be taken only orally requires active daily cooperation and compliance by the patient. In the event, this never transpired.

By June 1992 Dr Moss felt confident to recommend the removal of the Guardianship Order and to reduce the dosage of the depot medication still further.

Removal of Guardianship Order

Noting Dr Moss's firm opinion fifteen months earlier that the Guardianship Order was 'vital' until Andrew Robinson 'can demonstrate that he can take much more responsibility for himself', and that 'without regular supervision and medication there must remain a significant risk to members of the public', why did Dr Moss and Mr Steer feel so confident that the Order was no longer necessary? The decision is puzzling, particularly in the light of Dr Moss's own concerns in the clinical notes in September 1992, where he notes possible 'early warning symptoms' of impending breakdown. Furthermore, the following month, John Camus reported problems in getting Andrew to accept a full depot dose – he negotiated to give him only half. In February 1992, moreover, Andrew failed to attend his review appointment with Dr Moss. He had also, in early July 1992, received notice to quit his group home because of his failure to care for his room in a proper manner, and in early September he moved to a rented flat in Torquay owned by Mr and Mrs Hatsell. At the point of removal of the Order on 17 July 1992, Andrew was only very reluctantly accepting small doses of medication and was actively being ejected from his residence because of failure to cope.

While all three members of the clinical team were in agreement in June 1992 about the decision to remove the Guardianship Order, surely by late July alarm bells should have been ringing in all three of them, that the decision was precipitate and unwise? In defence of the decision, Dr Moss indicated to us that he knew Andrew Robinson had applied once more to the Tribunal for a discharge and that he had doubts that the Tribunal would support a further renewal in view of his relatively good mental state in June, his apparent compliance with medication and Dr Moss's judgment that there was no longer any danger to others. Mr Steer concurred with his view. He felt that there was no further benefit to be derived from the Guardianship Order. He further believed that, if the order had continued, 'the new found trust which Andrew had developed would have been irretrievably damaged and the benefits of the years of guardianship would have been limited at best'.

We are not convinced of the validity of this latter point and, in the light of Andrew's subsequent very rapid slide into the catastrophic relapse, which resulted in the tragedy under review, we regard the decision as having been ill-judged and unwise. We believe that the Guardianship Order could and should have been renewed indefinitely and, furthermore, that Andrew's appeal to the Tribunal would most likely have been unsuccessful, since the criteria for acceptance into Guardianship were more than adequately fulfilled.

It is interesting to note that local practice at that time in South Devon was to use Guardianship as a relatively short-term, time-limited order. Dr Moss made available to us a report he had compiled in June 1991 on the use of Guardianship Orders in South Devon between 1987 and 1991. There were a total of 34 orders made, 18 for patients over the age of 65 years, the majority of whom were suffering from dementia, and 16 for patients under 65 years, all except one of whom were suffering from schizophrenia or related psychoses. Dr Moss used Guardianship during this period rather more frequently than his general psychiatrist colleagues. Of the 34 orders, only 5 were renewed more than once, and 20 were never renewed after the initial period of Guardianship. The majority were simply allowed to lapse.

Dr Moss's report contains an interesting discussion of the usefulness of Guardianship in granting access by professionals to a patient who may not be complying with a care plan, and the report asks important questions about Guardianship and community-based treatment, which we address in Chapter XXI on the legal framework for community care. Dr Moss ends his report with this key question: 'If Guardianship Orders had been used at the appropriate point and properly, would there be less call for compulsory [community] treatment orders?' In Andrew Robinson's case, the question is whether, if the Guardianship Order had been continued, he would have persevered with treatment without compulsion. We think he probably would have.

Within a month of the Order being removed, Robert Steer had applied for and been appointed to a new post in Newton Abbot. Dr Moss too was planning to move on – he had been appointed to a consultant advisory post with a London-based mental health service development advisory organisation, and had resigned from his post as a full-time catchment area consultant psychiatrist, although he maintained links with the service. The team which had maintained Andrew Robinson effectively in the community (if not always 'well', at least out of the dangerous psychosis into which he could so quickly plunge) became in effect fragmented, leaving the key worker, John Camus, a state enrolled nurse, to soldier on alone, and without the backup of any legal powers in place to assist him. It was asking much too much of Mr Camus, even though he, above all, had established a working relationship with Andrew.

If the Guardianship Order had been continued, and if a new social worker and consultant psychiatrist had smoothly, and at the earliest opportunity replaced those leaving, it is at least probable that subsequent tragic events would have been avoided.

XIII. The Dénouement: Final Relapse in Mental Health, Autumn 1992 – 1 September 1993

> Lose this day loitering, 'twill be the same story
> To-morrow, and the next more dilatory;
> Each indecision brings its own delays.
> And days are lost lamenting o'er lost days.
> Are you in earnest? Seize this very minute!
> Boldness has genius, power, and magic in it,
> Only engage, and then the mind grows heated,
> Begin, and then the work will be completed.[*]

The period of relative stability over 30 months, produced by a combination of the Guardianship Order itself, the coordinated and constant care team of Dr Moss, Mr Camus and Mr Steer, and the regular receipt of medication, did not last. It was dismantled by the removal of the Guardianship Order, the breaking up of the care team and the inevitable ceasing of medication. The dismantling began at a review meeting on 2 June 1992, when a decision was made to lift the Guardianship Order. Dr Moss's note recorded: 'Discontinue Guardianship – but be prepared to reinstitute if need arises.' A letter from Rob Steer, Andrew's social worker, to the Social Services Area Manager on 21 July 1992 supported the decision: 'I believe that Andrew will continue to comply with the wishes of the community mental health team and has indicated that he is happy to carry on taking his medication.' Mr Steer concluded:

> I feel that the Guardianship Order has helped us to make some remarkable steps forward with Andrew and I feel that it is now an appropriate time to discharge the Order and give him more freedom. I intend to remain as Care Manager for him and John Camus in the Rehabilitation Team will be his community key worker. I have no hesitation in recommending that we discharge the Guardianship Order on Andrew. I believe that this action will even further improve

[*] John Austen [1793-1867], Faust Prologue for the Theatre, Manager's Speech.

his self-confidence and self-belief and lead to further improvements in his lifestyle.'

On 21 August 1992 the Guardianship Order was discharged. There were several other significant changes around this time. Andrew had been under notice since July 1992 to quit his accommodation for non-compliance with the house rules. On 7 September 1992 he moved from the rehabilitation hostel into a privately rented flat. There had also been a change in his medication. From December 1991 he had been receiving Clopixol 200 mg every two weeks. In June 1992 this was reduced to Clopixol 150 mg every two weeks, upon which Dr Moss commented at the time, 'we are getting near to the lowest acceptable limit'. On 22 September it was further reduced to 150 mg three-weekly. The care team itself was also changing. And Dr Moss noted in his letter of 23 September 1992 to Andrew's GP, Dr Speake: 'I should also note that both his social worker, Rob Steer, and I are likely to be moving onto other work in the next three months or so, and this break of continuity means that care should be taken in establishing new contacts, especially with the psychiatrist who takes my place. He will have a further review with us in four months' time.'

On 22 October 1992 John Camus visited Andrew with a view to administering his depot injection. He recorded: 'He was only willing to receive 75 mg instead of 150 ... have since discussed with Dr Moss who agrees that this was on the cards for some time and he feels it will not be long before Andrew refuses it altogether.'

Despite Dr Moss's apparent openness to the reinstitution of Guardianship, if the need arose, and his awareness of the need for careful management of the transition between care teams, and his view that Clopixol 150 mg two-weekly was close to the lowest acceptable limit, and Andrew was now well below that, no action was in fact taken. Dr Monteiro, who took over responsibility for Andrew from Dr Moss when the latter left, did not take up his post until 2 January 1993. In Dr Moss's written statement to the Inquiry he stated: 'An attempt to make an appointment with Dr Monteiro, my successor, was initiated on 17th December, probably after I had had a handing-over discussion with him (not recorded).'

Of the three key mental health professionals who had supported Andrew over the previous two years, only John Camus remained actively involved at this time. As an Enrolled Nurse, it was an unreasonable expectation for him to carry the responsibility for a mental health assessment, care planning and implementation. Mr

Camus, in theory, received supervision from Mr Les Grainger, a Registered Nurse and the Rehabilitation team leader at that time. Indeed, when in early November John Camus reported back to the Rehabilitation team his concerns about Andrew, Les Grainger carried out a home assessment. His note for 16 November 1992 read:

> Visited Andrew at home this pm. He is intending to go and stay at his parents' home whilst they are away in South Africa for some 3 months. Andrew appeared relaxed and was very friendly, imparted information freely and there was no evidence of any psychotic symptoms. He intends to arrange with J. Camus how he will continue with his depot when living at his parents house. I was impressed by the way in which Andrew presented himself today and I think that his time in Torquay has been beneficial for him.

This very reassuring assessment was in marked contrast to the picture conveyed by a letter from Andrew's father to Dr Moss, written on 29 October 1992:

> I think that I ought to let you know that my wife and I are not at all happy about Andrew, who has become very 'high' recently. This may not be immediately detectable in a short interview, but to us as parents it is only too clear ... This present condition may be partly due to the recent reduction in his medication, and partly due to the fact that we were unable/unwilling to give him £7000, to finance the publication of a book he has written! But his basic illness is the real cause – he continues to 'hear voices' (or however one describes it).

All the warning sounds were there, but they appear to have gone unheeded, even if they were heard.

Andrew moved into his parents' home in Sidmouth in November 1992. John Camus saw him once in Paignton, before visiting him there on 4 January 1993. On that occasion Andrew totally refused his depot injection, saying: 'He had reached the stage when he no longer needed a straitjacket.' Mr Camus continued the entry: 'I have to admit he appears better now than I have ever known him. He still has flights of ideas. His thoughts and what he says are far from conventional, but as he says, he is in control of this thinking and able to sort out what is real and what are his ideals and aspirations.' At this time Mr Camus was functioning with little or no clinical supervision. This is poignantly underlined by the fact that Mr Camus had taken his wife (who is an RMN) with him on the visit of 4 January 1993, 'because I wanted her to see how

Andrew was'. The absence of effective clinical supervision and enrolled status – and hence by John Camus's own admission his practical rather than theoretical orientation – contributed to an underestimation of the risks involved in Andrew's default from medication. The only other professional involved at this time was Dr Wride, a Community Medical Officer in psychiatry. He was consulted by Mr Camus, and arrangements were made for him to make an informal assessment of Andrew. This took place on 25 January 1993; the account of the assessment concluded:

> Andrew seems much more compliant and realistic in his outlook and view of his illness than I have previously seen. There is currently no evidence of any delusional thinking and he is quite happy to maintain regular contact with our new consultant.
> Plan – early appt to meet Dr Monteiro
> – no indication to force medication issue at present.

Worrying reports were, nevertheless, beginning to come through to the Rehabilitation team. Mrs Ingram, whom Andrew's parents had asked to look after the house and keep on eye on Andrew, became increasingly concerned about Andrew's behaviour. Her first contact with the Rehabilitation team was on 30 December 1992 when she rang to express her concerns. She rang John Camus on 8 February 1993, again greatly agitated. Again on 12 February 1993 she rang to inform him that Andrew was returning to Torquay. On 14 February 1993 a message was received, via the Out-of-hours Social Work Team, from the Sidmouth police that Andrew had been following an eleven-year-old boy who had been very worried by the experience. Urgent follow-up was requested. Andrew was offered an appointment with Dr Monteiro on 16 February 1993, which he did not keep. This was followed up with a joint home visit by Dr Wride and Mr Camus on 18 February 1993. In his record of the visit Dr Wride noted that Andrew was '... generally more agitated than when I saw him 2 weeks ago ... He protested that "the system" is out to get him and refused to consider seeing Dr Monteiro'. Dr Wride concluded: 'He is not in any way sectionable in his present state, but in view of his continued refusal to accept medication I suspect things will continue to deteriorate to the point that compulsory admission may be required.'

The picture was clearly emerging of a young man with a long history of severe psychotic disturbance, who had a demonstrable and, therefore, predictable pattern of deteriorating mental health

whenever medication was discontinued, whose behaviour was at-
tracting the attention and concern of a range of agencies, and who
was resisting engagement with the treatment packages that were
on offer. Alarm bells should have been ringing loud and clear. Dr
Monteiro, who as the RMO had responsibility for Andrew, had not
yet seen him. He did make a further attempt, by arranging a home
visit on 9 March 1993, but Andrew was out. Dr Monteiro did
eventually see Andrew briefly on 12 March 1993, when Andrew
'turned up unexpectedly at Culverhay', where Dr Monteiro was
seeing another patient. (The relevant note of that assessment has
been lost, along with a set of community notes.) Because Andrew
was at that time residing in an area that was the responsibility of
Dr McLaren, another Consultant Psychiatrist, and because he had
not yet been able to establish a relationship with Andrew, Dr
Monteiro decided to ask Dr McLaren to take over the care.

During March, Andrew's disturbed condition continued. On 3
March 1993 he was again preoccupied with killing. The record of a
Rehabilitation team meeting held on 9 March 1993 noted: 'John
wishes to visit Andrew at home. The team feels this may be
dangerous and we have suggested that he doesn't. If he doesn't
respond, John wants to visit him.'

In the face of mounting evidence of current disturbance in his
mental state, and a clear and predictable pattern of deterioration
with attendant increase in dangerousness, this period is characterised by a general agreement among the professionals involved
that there was a clear need for watchfulness. Effective intervention, however, was much less in evidence. In his statement to the
Inquiry, Mr Neil Lindup, a development worker for MIND in East
Devon, wrote: 'I certainly felt that he needed more professional help
than he seemed to be getting at the time and I did feel that
professionals should listen to carers and lay people such as myself.'
We heartily concur, on both points.

Against this backdrop, Dr McLaren assumed responsibility for
Andrew on 1 April 1993. Dr McLaren told us: 'I called for the
outpatient notes at an early stage but I didn't call for the inpatient
notes. I didn't get those until he was actually admitted.' Dr
Gillespie's assessment of Andrew in 1989, which said that he was
potentially very dangerous, and that no strategy should be resorted
to that involved the reduction or discontinuation of neuroleptics,
was recorded in the inpatient notes, but these were unavailable to
Dr McLaren at the time he took over responsibility for Andrew. We

asked Dr McLaren whether, if he had seen Dr Gillespie's assessment, he would have moved more speedily, to which he answered: 'I think I would have done, yes.' In the event, he arranged to see Andrew on 5 May 1993. In his written statement to the Inquiry, Dr McLaren explained: 'This was a routine appointment as, given the information available to me at the time, I did not regard the situation as urgent.' Andrew failed to keep the appointment of 5 May, just as he had failed to keep an appointment with the Torquay Rehabilitation team on 29 April. A further complication at this time was that, although medical responsibility for Andrew had been transferred, the community mental health team at Torquay, with which Dr McLaren was linked, was unaware of this. When, therefore, a request to transfer community care came from John Camus at the Paignton team, to Mike Gagg from the Torquay Rehabilitation team, Mr Gagg expressed reservations about the wisdom of such a transfer while Andrew was apparently far from stable. When questioned about his reluctance to take over Andrew's care, Mr Gagg said: 'I appear to have been aware that Andrew Robinson was in an acute phase, and that I feel very strongly that it is a bad time to refer somebody to the Rehabilitation team.'

This apparent confusion about who was responsible was current at the time Andrew was missing appointments with the Rehabilitation team and with Dr McLaren. On 6 May 1993 there was a meeting of the Paignton team that involved Dr Moss, who was covering a period of leave for Dr Monteiro, and Mr Gagg who was providing senior nursing support for the team in the absence of Mr Grainger who had left early in the year. Andrew was discussed at that meeting, and following it Mr Gagg wrote to Dr McLaren:

> Stuart, Dr Moss was present at Culverhay and was adamant after hearing the team's concerns that we should act, as the three important people in Andrew's care have left. They are Dr Moss, Les Grainger and Rob Steer – social worker now at Laurels. I leave it to you to discuss with GP and acute team how to progress.

There is a postscript: 'There is apparently an application for a firearms licence on his table.' In a letter written on the same day (6 May 1993) to Joy Wiltshire, the Culverhay manager, Mr Gagg repeated that 'it is impossible for me to assume responsibilities for a man I've not met, especially at a time of crisis and when medical responsibility is unclear'. Mr Gagg added that while Andrew was 'apparently in need of inpatient treatment, I would suggest an admission to the Edith Morgan Centre be considered'. This letter was copied widely, because as Mr Gagg explained to us: 'I was concerned. I was concerned about safety. I felt that people were possibly expecting me to do something and I wanted all those people to be aware that I wasn't.'

By mid-May 1993 Andrew's parents were so concerned that they wrote on 14 May forcefully to the Director of Devon Social Services: 'He decided not to have any more depot injections in November and has steadily deteriorated ... As parents we are deeply distressed, and with his past history feel this can only end in tragedy if he continues to go without medication ... If nothing is done soon and anything happens to our son I shall hold you responsible ....' Two days previously, Dr McLaren had written to the Robinsons offering them an appointment on 9 June 1993. That interview went ahead. On the same day Andrew turned up at EMC to visit John Camus. He was admitted on a section 4 of the Mental Health Act 1983. This was rapidly converted to a section 3 admission. In his medical recommendation Dr McLaren wrote: 'He is showing evidence of a relapse of paranoid schizophrenia .... From the history, he poses a major physical threat to others when in relapse.'

This admission took place exactly thirteen months after the review meeting at which the decision was made, in principle, to remove the Guardianship Order, but leaving open the possibility of reinstatement, should the need arise. Two and a half months later, August 1992, the Guardianship Order was lifted. Two months after that, Andrew started refusing his full medication, at the same time as his parents were expressing renewed concerns. By January 1993, Andrew was refusing all his medication. Dr Moss, Mr Steer and Mr Grainger had all moved on, and Mr Camus was left as the only constant professional. From January to June 1993, amid mounting concern from carers and family, Andrew was seen only once, and then only briefly, by his RMO. His main contact was an Enrolled Nurse who heroically maintained an excellent relationship with Andrew but should not have been expected to take responsibility for undertaking a full mental state assessment. Everything in late 1992 and early 1993 pointed to the dire need to reinstate the highly successful Guardianship Order. That it was not reinstated was a mistake, due in large part to the change in personnel in mental health services.

The period from January to June 1993 was one of fluctuating professional concern, with a measure of inactivity that does not square with the information readily available to inform a more proactive risk-assessment and intervention. The consequence of this period of inactivity was that Andrew's psychosis had time to ripen into a full blown paranoid state, with a complete absence of insight. It was in this parlous state of mental ill-health that he began his final inpatient admission at EMC.

When Andrew Robinson was compulsorily admitted to EMC on 9 June 1993 he was placed in the ECA. He had his first escorted leave to the main unit three days later. He was reported in the nursing notes: 'Not happy about being here, but no point in running away.' Later that same day, he had 3 hours unescorted leave on the main unit. During his period on ECA he was agitated, restless, described as grimacing and constantly scratching his head. His thoughts remained 'very jumbled and much of his time was spent writing compulsively on scraps of paper'. By 14 June he was adjudged to be sufficiently settled to be transferred to the main unit. On transfer, John Camus recorded: 'On the surface he is quite calm and keeping it together. Underneath he is quite disturbed.' Over the next few days Andrew was described variously as very restless, with disturbed and bizarre thought content; 'obviously tormented'; 'very disturbed at a lower level'. Despite this presentation, the nursing note for 21 June recorded that he 'went to town shopping'. There is no corresponding entry in the medical notes for that day, nor was there any reference to his absence from EMC in the record of the ward round held by Dr McLaren on 24 June. Although his depot medication had been reinstituted, along with oral psychotropic drugs, there was little evidence of his psychosis subsiding. Dr McLaren's record of the ward round was: 'Remains prominently deluded with strong persecutory ideas.' On 29 June the medical notes recorded: 'Remains deluded, expressing persecutory ideas regarding people wanting to kill him.' This picture is reflected in the nursing notes, although the entry for 29 June added: 'Seen by Dr McLaren. Feels that medication is gradually working.' Andrew's obsessional writing continued throughout this period.

There are two entries in the nursing notes for 3 July. The first read: 'Phoned his landlady at 8 am and arranged to go and collect money. He did this and returned an hour later. No problems on unit.' The second entry, made later that day by John Camus, read: 'Andrew appeared very uptight early afternoon, said he felt "caged-in" – was given permission to go out – returned at 7 pm much more

relaxed – no extra meds given.' In oral evidence Mr Camus was
asked by Miss Davies:

> Q. Who gave him permission to go out?
> A. I can't be sure. I would have to assume that it would have been
>   whoever was in charge of the Torquay team at that time.
> Q. When you say 'In charge of the Torquay team', would that be
>   within the Edith Morgan Centre?
> A. Yes.
> Q. Would that be a nurse or a doctor?
> A. That would have been the charge nurse/sister, who was in charge
>   of the shift at that time.

This evidence was given in a manner that demonstrated what
was an everyday occurrence in the pattern of life at EMC. Dr
McLaren, who was the only person who could authorise leave,
denied knowing that any leave had been granted, or that Andrew
ever had left the unit, except for two occasions when it was reported
to him that Andrew had absconded – once on 6 July and again on
31 August 1993.

The fact that Andrew was leaving the unit on what was, by his
own admission, an almost daily basis was not, however, kept a
secret. The nursing notes erratically recorded, in a matter of fact
way, a selection of trips out. The Care Plan of 6 July identified as
one of Andrew's problems: 'He is continually leaving the unit
without prior knowledge of the team.' Even the terms in which this
is couched indicate that the problem was perceived, not that Andrew was leaving the unit, but that the staff had no prior notice of
his absence.

On 6 July, when he was discovered missing from the unit, the
police were notified. When Andrew returned independently to the
unit, two hours later, he appeared 'more settled and appropriate in
behaviour'. Dr McLaren was informed about this unauthorised
absence during the ward round later that day, although there was
no mention of the episode in the medical notes. What was recorded
by Dr McLaren was an assessment that Andrew was 'still psychotic
... spending lots of money on printing an article with bizarre
content'.

> Also took overdose of tablets for modified narcosis. Not sleeping at
> all. Wandering around, verbally aggressive, possible physical ag-
> gression. Plan: 1. Return to ECA. 2. Change Depixol to Clopixol 300
> mgs 3. ? long term – ?Cypress but will need longer assessment prior.

When Andrew was readmitted to ECA later that day, the entry in the nursing notes gave the reason as being, 'he's become over-stimulated whilst out on the main unit'. While in the ECA, Andrew continued to have periods of agitation, interspersed with periods of withdrawal. The printing firm, to whom he had taken his manuscript, telephoned the unit, complaining that they were receiving frequent calls from Andrew and wanted them stopped. On 8 July, following that call, Andrew was instructed to make no further calls to the printers; eventually the calls ceased. The calls were replaced, however, by letters. After representation to EMC, these too stopped.

At the ward round on 13 July it was decided that Andrew was ready to return to the main unit, 'with strict boundaries, clear programme'. There is no record of how that was to be translated into practice. Both nursing and medical notes recorded the persistence of delusional ideas, but improvement in mental state was noted. Periods of leave from the unit continued to be noted in the nursing records. On 18 July Andrew 'went out with his mother this afternoon for a short while'. On 23 July he 'went home with key worker for short while this pm'. (That was the same day as Andrew was seen on the ward round by Dr McLaren.) The notes recorded a view that 'secure provision not indicated'. But they make no reference to periods of leave from the unit, escorted or unescorted, planned, or even having taken place.

The remainder of Andrew's stay in EMC followed much the same pattern as the first six weeks. At times, he presented himself as restless, agitated; at other times, verbally aggressive. At yet other times he appeared withdrawn, over-sedated and depressed. Throughout, his thought disorder was marked, although there were times when he appeared to be able to control the expression of disturbance better than at others. In response to his presentation of over-sedation, on 10 August Zuclopenthixol – oral medication – was discontinued. His depot medication remained at Clopixol 300 mg, 2 weeks. Andrew's unauthorised absences from the unit continued unabated.

Mrs Hatsell, his landlady at the time, told us that, during this period, she thought Andrew was let out of EMC on a 'daily basis'. 'I saw him almost as often then as when I saw him before.' Mr Camus, when asked if he was aware that Andrew was leaving the unit on numerous occasions, as described by Mrs Hatsell, told us:

'Yes, I think that we were all aware that Andrew left the unit on a number of occasions.'

On 25 August 1993 Andrew once again left the unit, without authorisation. The fact went unrecorded. It was on that occasion that he made the purchase of the kitchen knife with which he assaulted Georgina Robinson on 1 September 1993.

From 9 June until 1 September 1993 Andrew was a detained patient in EMC. As Dr McLaren noted in his medical recommendation written on 9 June: 'He is showing evidence of a relapse of paranoid schizophrenia ... poses a major physical threat to others when in relapse.' This was an accurate risk assessment. Yet, for all that, there was little evidence of its impact on Andrew's treatment package. Throughout the 3-month period he remained thought-disordered, with evidence of significant disturbance. Even when Andrew was more able to control manifestation of that disturbance, the paranoia persisted. There appear to have been two ways in which a presentation of agitation was dealt with by Andrew's care team. Andrew was either given a spell in the ECA, or he was 'given permission' to go into town with or without an escort. By any standards, the latter would seem to be a wholly inadequate response. Granted that it is very easy to be wise after the event, it would still seem that the granting of unescorted leave to a patient with Andrew's history – who was judged to be a significant threat when in psychotic relapse, and who was exhibiting evidence of a very live psychosis – was a very ill-advised course of action. Leave to a detained patient is dealt with in Chapter XV.

The only other issue to be picked up here relates to the paucity of multi-disciplinary care planning for Andrew during his admission. There is mention, from time to time, of establishing a structured programme for Andrew. But nowhere is the content of, or the engagement with, that programme in evidence. On 13 July, when the decision was taken to transfer Andrew from ECA to the main unit, it was on the understanding that there would be 'strict boundaries'. From the nursing notes there was no evidence of any drawing of boundary lines, or of putting them into practice. It may be that the notes are an inadequate reflection of the multi-disciplinary care planning and implementation that in fact did go on in relation to Andrew. The picture that emerges from the documentary evidence is, however, that of a very disturbed young man who was allowed to drift about aimlessly in and out of the unit, and for whom the only focused treatment lay in medication. That there would be difficulty in engaging Andrew in treatment activities is understandable. That there was apparently no attempt to do so is incomprehensible. Even with a more robust approach to treatment, the outcome on 1 September 1993 might have been the same. But equally it might not.

XIV. Judgment on the Fatal Event

Vision is the art of seeing things invisible.[*]

'Not every human disaster' – as Dr Adrian Grounds reminds us in his stimulating contribution to the publication accompanying this report[1] – 'can be predicted and prevented.' That presupposes that many, if not most, can be. We have therefore asked ourselves: was the fatal incident of 1 September 1993 predictable and/or preventable? We have posed the question in that form because we perceive that if the specific event could not have been predicted, nevertheless it might still have been prevented. If it had been predicted, it would or should, of course, more than likely have been prevented.

There is the wider question whether, putting to one side the event immediately surrounding the fatal event of 1 September 1993, it was predictable that at any time after June 1978 Andrew Robinson, if and when he was ever again in a psychotic state of mind, would violently assault another person (specifically, a young woman) or commit suicide. We consider that wider question first, relying heavily on the criteria for assessing risk suggested by Dr Grounds.

Predictability

We, in common with all similar inquiries, have been suitably conscious of the need to guard against resort to hindsight. As Dr Grounds informed us, there is an added factor in the eyes of a clinician in retrospectively assessing the risk. When reflecting on the history of someone who has committed in the past a serious offence, one is apt to focus selectively on factors which appear to have contributed to the outcome. Dr Grounds put it neatly in four propositions, which we quote:

First, the assessment of risk involves consideration of three different

[*] Jonathan Swift, *Thoughts on Various Subjects* (1711).
[1] J.H.M. Crichton (ed.) *Psychiatric Patient Violence: Risk and Response* (1995) London: Gerald Duckworth & Co. (p. 47, citing the NHS Executive document, 1994, paras 26-28).

components, namely an outcome (e.g. an offence), the likelihood of the outcome, and a time frame. Secondly, predictions of the future can be wrong in two ways: there are false positive outcomes – harm occurs when it was predicted it would not; and false negative outcomes: harm does not occur when it was predicted that it would. In decisions about release or detention of patients both errors can have adverse consequences. Thirdly, in clinical assessment there is the danger of hindsight bias. In the context of a Public Inquiry, this is an important point. When looking back at the history of someone who has committed a serious offence, we selectively focus on the factors which appear to have contributed to the outcome. This can make an event that is statistically unlikely – an offence with a low base rate – look highly probable or even inevitable. This in turn can lead us to overestimate future dangerousness. Fourthly, clinical assessment is not primarily about making an accurate prediction but about making informed, defensible decisions about dangerous behaviour. The test is not one of accuracy, but how defensible the decision is in terms of social realities and current scientific knowledge.

This is an echo of the salutary warning, given many years ago by the late Dr Peter Scott, that 'dangerousness is a dangerous concept'. What is demanded is not an assessment of dangerousness, but an acknowledgment of the relation of risk-assessment to management strategy adapting timeously to the patient's changing mental condition. This approach was most compellingly put to us by Dr Gallwey in respect of management's response to any risk-assessment. Exchanges between him and Mr Thorold spelt out the need of clinicians and managers to be more than ordinarily watchful whenever a detained patient with a record of violent behaviour lapses into a psychotic condition:

Q. I would like to ask you, as a specialist in assessing patients of this kind, how did you come to look at the risk that this kind of ideation might translate into action?

A. Well, there is always a problem with any ideation. You cannot say what the risk is except in terms of previous behaviour, response to treatment, and residual sanity really, including insight. There is not any way of predicting who is going to live out their sadistic feelings or homicidal feelings, and particularly in psychosis, of course, it is pretty well unpredictable.

Q. So when you say it is difficult to predict, are you thinking more about people in their non-psychotic phases?

A. I am saying that when somebody is psychotic and they have homicidal or sadistic ideation as part and parcel of the psychosis, then you really cannot predict whether they are going to live it out or not, except in terms of past behaviour. In other words, the worrying thing about this patient was that he had lived it out, so far as he had gone to somebody with a shotgun, and my understanding of it was, whatever he said about it, that it was in fact a potential homicide, so that was very worrying.

Clearly our task was to see whether that violence was a factor of his psychosis, and if it was, did the psychosis settle satisfactorily, and if it did then the violence should go because if it was a factor of the psychosis the danger should go and the psychosis remits. Of course, some patients are violent in their personalities and then when the psychosis settles the violence may get worse and the risk greater.

Although it is really quite a simple way of approaching these cases, he fell into the first category, in so far as his psychosis remitted he became more and more amenable and pleasant and cooperative and the really rather charming and pleasant side to him came to the fore. That was very reassuring in so far as one felt that provided his psychosis was controlled and kept an eye on then he should be safe.

and later Dr Gallwey summarised his view that, when in a psychotic state, Andrew Robinson had to be treated by management as though it was dealing with a dangerous patient:

Q. Before we go to precise terms, is it possible to select out the headline messages that you would convey back, or would want to have conveyed to any subsequent reader of a discharge report, based on the time he was at the Butler with you?

A. Yes.

Q. That when psychotic he really could be very dangerous?

A. Well, when psychotic he had been dangerous and therefore it had to be presumed he might be in the future. It is not to say that ...

Q. You would have to make that presumption?

A. You would have to make the presumption that there was a degree of unknown dangerousness and that he was in that sense unpredictable, yes.

Q. You would have to be on your guard?

A. Yes.

Q. That he could, even when not psychotic, be quite dangerous but that might be dependent on the circumstances then arising and could be guarded against to some degree by alert observation?

A. I don't think I felt he was dangerous when he was not psychotic, no.

Looking back at the index offence of 3 June 1978, in its full implications, as we have done, one must conclude that it was a very serious offence that was all too repeatable if the same mental and situational ingredients were present – i.e. a psychotic disorder with strong homicidal ideations directed towards an identifiable female in his life. The essential ingredient of psychosis would always be present so long as Andrew was not kept indefinitely on supervised medication. That was the view in 1980 of Dr Udwin who, with his colleagues at Broadmoor, so successfully treated Andrew that he could be released on a conditional discharge within 2½ years at the Special Hospital. It was a view confirmed a decade later by Dr Gallwey on discharging Andrew at the end of 1989 from the RSU back to EMC. In answer to the question, 'so it was your view at the end of the period of the assessment that in order to prevent him becoming psychotic once more it was essential to keep him on medication?', Dr Gallwey replied: 'Yes.' And, when presented with the full picture of the 1978 event and Andrew's horrendous scribblings of 1989, Drs Orr, Moss and McLaren all acknowledged a heightened sense of the risk of future violent behaviour from Andrew. The problem that arose in this case was that, except for those directly involved with Andrew's mental health in and around 1978, and Dr Gallwey in 1989, no one had a full appreciation of the nature of the index offence. Had all the clinicians been made aware of the 1978 event, we think – without having to reach for our retrospectoscope – that they would have concluded that Andrew presented a high risk, if not adequately medicated under supervision. We think this, having full regard to the fact that the great majority of seriously mentally ill people who are in the community are not violent. Andrew was, we conclude, decidedly one of the minority.

It is not just the 1978 offence that provides the clue to Andrew being a high risk. The assessment of risk, which must be grounded in history, is not to be confined to the single event of serious violence. Evidence of repetition of the context of the earliest incident in which harm was inflicted should be viewed. To that end, records must be examined in detail to see if bouts of violent behaviour occur. Of those there were numerous occasions, both when Andrew was with his family and when he was hospitalised. It is only too apparent to us that insufficient risk assessment was undertaken during the final episode of Andrew's mental illness leading up to and including his compulsory admission to EMC in June – August 1993. Had there been a proper assessment of risk of further violent behaviour, it did not take a visionary to see what might happen if Andrew was not kept under close scrutiny while hospitalised and, if discharged to the community in the future, kept under supervised medication.

It was predictable that one day Andrew Robinson, if he was not maintained on medication under proper supervision, would kill, probably a young woman with whom he had entertained some emotional relationship. But Georgina Robinson was a complete stranger to Andrew Robinson; it was entirely fortuitous that she unhappily became the victim of the assault. Andrew's ideation was so uninhibited, when psychotic, that his main focus on women with whom he had been closely associated was irrelevant on 1 September 1993. In the summer of 1993, Andrew Robinson was too loose a cannon (for modernists, an unguided missile) for anyone in sight to be regarded as safely off target. Steps could and should have been taken to prevent the eventuality of some violent incident.

We have indicated in our report that, way back in September 1986, the conditional discharge should not have been lifted. We think that the Guardianship Order should have remained in force after 1992, under the supervision of a fresh team to succeed Dr Moss, Mr Steer and Mr Camus; and we think that Andrew should have been 'sectioned' much earlier than June 1993. None of these sensible steps could foreseeably have prevented the incident of 1 September 1993. But could the incident, nevertheless, have been prevented as a result of other practical steps, taken as ordinary precautions in an inpatient psychiatric facility in respect of a detained patient?

Preventability

The assault on Georgina Robinson was the direct consequence of three linked events: (i) Andrew Robinson's unauthorised absence from EMC during most of the week preceding the fatal incident on 1 September 1993; (ii) while absent from EMC, Andrew's unhindered purchase on 25 August 1993 of a dangerous weapon, a kitchen knife, from the Co-op in Torquay; and (iii) Andrew's possession of the kitchen knife, undisclosed to and undiscovered by the staff at EMC between the time of Andrew's return on 31 August 1993 and the assault at 4 o'clock the next afternoon. Had Andrew's absence from EMC been authorised, there would be a real question whether any authorisation of leave of absence (with or without an escort) would have been reasonable, and whether the acquisition of a dangerous weapon in the hands of a high-risk patient was foreseeable. But the two absences from EMC – the absence on 25 August 1993 without the knowledge of staff, and the leave granted by a senior nurse on 28 August 1993 – were unlawful. The former occurred as a result of a lax policy at EMC, whereby patients generally were able to move in and out of the hospital, without let or hindrance from anyone or anything. The latter resulted from a breach of section 17, Mental Health Act 1983. Andrew could not lawfully have been allowed to leave EMC without the specific and exclusive authority of his RMO, Dr McLaren, who was unaware of Andrew's request (and in any event, would have refused leave). Had Andrew Robinson been denied – as he should have been – both the freedom to go to Torquay on 25 August and to wander around in London and Torquay for 3 days, from 28 to 31 August, Georgina almost certainly would not have been fatally assaulted by Andrew on 1 September 1993. Georgina Robinson's death was in that sense preventable, the responsibility for which lies with the Trust's management and staff of EMC.

We mention two other aspects of preventive action relevant to the incident on 1 September 1993. First, the absence of any policy towards searching the person and belongings of a detained patient returning from absence without leave. Mental health units should develop a clear policy on when a personal search will be carried out. An agreement to grant leave could, for example, be made on the explicit condition that non-compliance with the terms of leave may be followed by a search, if staff have cause for concern that harmful objects may have been brought into the ward.

The second area of prevention concerns the delay which took place in coming to Georgina's aid as a result of there being no patient or staff alarm system. The Trust submitted a report to us about the security arrangements within EMC which considered in some depth the question of whether to instal further alarm systems. The final decision on whether to purchase a new alarm system for the unit has been delayed until the report of our Inquiry has been received. The Trust's view, however, is that such expenditure would be inappropriate, given the limited life-span of the present building. The matter has been investigated and discussed; estimates from three different companies have been obtained; the estimated cost of installation is not insubstantial at around £20,000. Furthermore, the Trust has made several changes already to ensure that the main areas where incidents take place are adequately covered, and we concur with its view that a short-term heavy investment in EMC is not warranted.

We understand that a unit-wide location alarm system has been included in the design brief for the new building and, while this will improve the safety of staff by ensuring they can reach an alarm quickly, it will not necessarily resolve the problems for patients who need to raise an alarm. We think it is essential that patients, who are as much at risk of violent incidents as members of staff, should have ready access to incident alarms. A fear has been expressed that a minority of patients might abuse the alarms – and it is true that fire alarms are on occasion rung for reasons other than a fire – but visible and easy-to-reach incident alarms should cause no more trouble than fire alarms and would add substantially to the feeling of security and also to the real safety of patients. We hope that the Trust will instal a system which gives equal comfort to staff and patients alike.

Part D

General Issues

XV. Lawless Absenteeism

Is it not a pleasant tribute to the medical profession that by and large it has been able to manage its relations with its patients ... without the aid of lawyers and lawmakers?*

As a detained patient in EMC from 9 June 1993 onwards, Andrew Robinson should not have been allowed to leave EMC (or at least not the hospital grounds) without permission grantable exclusively by his RMO, Dr Stuart McLaren. While the staff could hardly stop him leaving EMC – because, most of the time, they did not know his whereabouts and there was no check on his (or any other patients') movements – he sometimes did seek and obtain ostensible permission from senior nursing staff to be away from the District General Hospital on which EMC is sited. But he often did leave without permission and regularly went wandering around in Torquay.

He appeared to be absent, without leave, on 25 August 1993, during which day he purchased the weapon (a Prestige kitchen knife) with which he fatally wounded Georgina Robinson a week later. But he was specifically given leave by a senior nurse on 28 August to be away in Torquay for the day; he failed to return that evening, and was absent without leave until 31 August. How did it come about that no notice, let alone attention was paid to the provisions of the law prescribing the method for granting Andrew Robinson, a detained patient, leave of absence? To answer that question, which supplied a vital circumstance surrounding the death of Georgina Robinson, we first indicate the state of the law and good practice and consider what changes, if any, need to be made; secondly, we set out the evidence of the state of the knowledge of staff; thirdly, we consider where the responsibility lies for the failure of EMC to give effect at any time to the legal provision in the Mental Health Act 1983. Fourthly, we advert to the allied case of Stephen Hext.

---

* Lord Devlin in his Lloyd Roberts Lecture 'Medicine and the Law' (1960) to the Medical Society of London, in *Samples of Lawmaking* (1962), p. 103.

The present law

The RMO may grant leave of absence to any compulsory patient under section 17 of the Mental Health Act 1983, but if the patient is under a restriction order the permission of the Home Secretary is required. Since it opened in 1986, EMC have admitted only two restricted patients, so that it is unlikely that the limitation on the RMO's power was ever in general contemplation. Leave can be given for a special occasion (a family funeral or wedding) or for a definite period (a day out shopping or a weekend at home) or indefinitely. It can be extended without bringing the patient back to hospital. But it can also be revoked at any time if the RMO thinks it is necessary in the interests of the patient's own health or safety, or for the protection of other people. Notice of revocation and recall must be in writing and addressed either to the patient or to the person in charge of him. Leave can be subject to whatever conditions the RMO thinks necessary in the patient's interests, or to protect him. This may include staying in another hospital, living with another person (usually at the patient's home) or attending a clinic for treatment. The patient remains liable to detention and, hence, can be obliged to accept medical treatment, subject to the usual statutory safeguards. The effect of this is that the patient can be apprehended the moment he becomes absent without leave, rather than if and when he fails to return to hospital. An important condition to be considered when granting leave of absence is whether the patient should be away from the hospital, unescorted or not.

Legislative history of section 17

The legal provisions for permitting a patient to be absent for such period as may be thought fit, for the benefit of his health, are traceable back to the Care and Treatment of Lunatics Act, 8 & 9 VICT. c.100 (1845). Section 86 of that Act provided:

> ... it shall be lawful for the Proprietor or Superintendent of any licensed House or of any Hospital, with the Consent in Writing of any Two of the Commissioners ... to send or take, under proper Control, any Patient to any specified Place for any definite Time for the Benefit of his Health: Provided always, nevertheless, that before any such Consent as aforesaid shall be given by any Commissioners or Visitors the Approval in Writing of the Person who signed the

Order for the Reception of such Patient, or by whom the past Payment on account of such Patient was made, shall be produced to such Commissioners or Visitors, unless they shall, on cause being shown, dispense with the same.

Section 17 of the Lunacy (Amendment) Act 1855 amended the law to make the consent of the Committee of Management of a hospital sufficient to authorise a patient being sent to any specified place for any definite time. And section 38 of the Lunacy (Amendment) Act 1862 extended the authorisation 'to permit any patient to be absent from such hospital upon trial; for such period as may be thought fit'. That language found its way into section 55 of the Lunacy Act 1890. Apart from authorisation by a Commissioner or Committee of Management of a hospital, by sub-section (7) of section 55 'the medical officer of a hospital may, of his own authority, permit any patient to be absent from the hospital for a period not exceeding forty-eight hours'. Regulations 4 and 5 of the Mental Treatment Rules 1948 and Regulations 95 and 96 of the Mental Deficiency Regulations 1948 similarly provided for 'leave of absence' to be granted in writing to the patient for a limited period. A form for granting permission was prescribed in the Rules.

Section 39 of the Mental Health Act 1959 (apart from one minor amendment in the 1983 Act) was the immediate forerunner of section 17 of the 1983 Act. It enacted the recommendations of the Royal Commission (the Percy Commission) on the law relating to mental illness and mental deficiency 1954-1957 (Cmnd. 169) which considered elaborating the circumstances whereby a patient should remain under compulsory powers but allowed to be away from the hospital. Paragraph 458 (p. 155) of the Report described the instance where patients need to be transferred from the hospital to another hospital and community care. It added:

> Patients also sometimes go home to their families for a week-end or a longer holiday, or to a holiday home, with the expectation of returning to the hospital afterwards. Sometimes patients are sent to live outside the hospital to see how they get on, before the doctors decide whether they should be discharged or not; if they do not succeed in adapting themselves to life outside, they may need to return to the hospital for further treatment or training. In other cases the doctors may decide that the patient can continue to live outside the hospital if suitable community care is ensured, and, in some cases, if some powers of control are still exercised over the patient. Patients who have been receiving community care under compulsory control also sometimes need to be admitted to hospital.

and in para. 469 it said:

> It is generally agreed that it should be possible for patients to be away from hospital for short periods, for a holiday or for a period of treatment in another hospital or for any other reason approved by the medical superintendent, without breaking the existing compulsory powers and without any cumbersome procedure when the patient leaves or returns.

Accordingly the Percy Commission recommended (para. 477, p. 161) that a detained patient should be able to leave the hospital at any time and for any purpose with the approval of the responsible doctor, without the compulsory powers being lifted. There has never been any authorisation for granting leave of absence by nursing staff.

Code of Practice for the 1983 Act

The Code of Practice recites the main provisions of the 1983 Act and amplifies (but does not extend) the law.[1] The decision to grant leave cannot be delegated to a professional colleague such as a doctor in training or a member of the nursing staff (para. 20.4.a(i)). The decision should be made 'after necessary consultation' with clinical staff caring for and treating the patient. Para 20.2 of the Code states that the patient should be fully involved in the decision to grant leave and must be asked to consent to any consultation with others (e.g. relatives, professionals in community care) thought necessary before leave is granted. The patient 'should be able to demonstrate to his professional carers that he is likely to cope outside the hospital'. Leave is not required if the patient is kept within the hospital grounds.

Shortly after the appearance of the 1st edition of the Code of Practice, which the Secretary of State was bound by statute to prepare and lay before Parliament for the guidance of practitioners in the mental health field, further advice was published by the Mental Health Act Commission in its 4th biennial report, 1989-1991 (published in December 1991). The Commission said at para. 9.7:

> Leave of absence from hospital under s. 17 is often a major compo-

---

[1] We reproduce as an annex to this chapter para. 20, indicating the changes made between the 1st edition (December 1989) and 2nd edition (August 1993).

nent of rehabilitation programmes. Such leave may cover periods of absence from a single night up to six months. Short term absences of only a few hours also feature extensively in treatment plans and are sometimes regarded as a form of parole arranged at ward level in the hospital. The Act, however, describes leave of absence without mention of its duration whilst its granting is the prerogative solely of the responsible medical officer. The occurrence of any untoward incident during absence from hospital could raise the question of its planning and authorisation. On the other hand the requirement to obtain responsible medical officer agreement for every activity outside the hospital would seriously curtail any patient's involvement in the social programme and other rehabilitative activities which are often arranged at short notice by ward staff. The recommendation of the Commission is that all absences from hospital should be regarded as constituting leave with a need for responsible medical officer authorisation but that such leave should be agreed periodically, the weekly multi-disciplinary conference being an ideal occasion, with a written statement of the maximum licence that is granted for a defined period and with any related conditions. Staff implementing the treatment programme would then be free to arrange absences from hospital within the known limits and without need to obtain further more detailed authorisations.

That advice did not appear to have percolated to the management and staff of EMC. We digress to say, however, that the Commissioners who visited EMC annually never alluded in writing either to the existence of section 17, or to the fact that there appeared to be total non-compliance with the law, the Code, or the Commission's own advice. In their report of the visit of 4 May 1990, the Commissioners stated that they 'understood that policies, procedures and guide notes are being produced and distributed in the Edith Morgan Centre', no reference being made specifically to leave of absence practices. The Commission visit in February 1991 made no reference to the issue. Likewise, the visit report in February 1992 was silent on the topic, although it has to be said, in vindication, that there were no detained patients in the hospital. The report from the February 1993 visit did peripherally touch on the point. It said that EMC and other units in the hospital were visited 'and all the detained patients not on section 17 leave seen'.

No questions appeared on that occasion to be asked about the operation by staff of section 17, but the report tartly observed that 'there appeared to be minimum preparation for the [Commission's] visit and the impression gained was one of total confusion. Although there were only three detained patients, it was difficult for

Commissioners to obtain their records and even more difficult to locate members of staff. The records, when they did appear, were disorganised ... It was difficult to make sense of them ...' By contrast, all the required documentation was readily available in one of the other units, and the documentation relating to the Mental Health Act was in 'Excellent order and the medical records officer and staff were congratulated'. But nothing emerged in the Commission's report to indicate compliance with section 17. To criticisms directed at EMC, the Trust responded on 21 June 1993 (twelve days after Andrew Robinson's final admission) 'that the comments of Commissioners have been noted. The importance of statutory documents has now been reinforced to all staff. Medical cards and patients records are now the subject of regular audit.'

The Commission's visit in February 1994, following on both the circumstances of Georgina Robinson's death and the suicide of Stephen Hext on 17 December 1993, was sharply focused on section 17 leave. The Commission's report highlighted the deficiency in this regard, by drawing attention to the law and advising that 'a policy should be prepared, based on the requirements of the Code of Practice'. The Chairman of the Psychiatric Consultants' Committee, Dr John Lambourn, responded on 22 June 1994: 'We now have a fully agreed policy covering leave of absence which is totally in line with the Commission's "recommendation".'

For tardiness in instituting a policy for granting patients' leave of absence, and for failing to prescribe the appropriate documentation whereby leave is granted, responsibility must be borne by the South Devon Healthcare Trust. The MHAC must share the blame in not having pointed up the deficiency of any document indicating the Trust's policy and procedure for implementing the leave of absence provisions. It has taken two tragic incidents to alert the managers of an inpatient facility containing detained patients, and the patients' statutory watchdog body, to an important issue of security for patients, staff and the public. The Commission should have been alive to this aspect in its annual visits; and the Trust (since it came into existence in 1991) through its senior management, should have attended to all aspects of security. The clinicians (consultants and nursing staff) cannot be blamed for the failures of management. Their own lack of knowledge or awareness of the law and practice is a matter to which we now turn.

Staff knowledge of section 17

In its written evidence to us, the management of South Devon Healthcare Trust conceded that 'it is now accepted that there were occasions when the Code of Practice was breached'. Parenthetically, we observe that even in that, somewhat grudging concession, it is not fully appreciated that the breaches are violations of section 17 of the 1983 Act, for which the Code of Practice, after 1989, merely spelt out the law and good practice in non-legalistic language.

The Trust further admitted that 'it had no separate document on this issue, although the requirement to adhere to all aspects of the Code of Practice had been drawn to the attention of all mental health professionals when it was circulated'. That omission is being swiftly repaired, as we have noted in the response to the Mental Health Act Commission. (We have been shown a near final draft of a comprehensive procedure. In its final form it should be thoroughly reviewed at the next visit – in February 1995 – of the Mental Health Act Commission.)

The written evidence went on to explain, although commendably not to excuse, how the situation of ignorance of the law arose. It said:

In large mental hospitals with extensive grounds, <u>it was common practice for the staff to allow patients to go to and from other therapeutic and social activities without resort to the granting of leave</u>. Where the levels of observation set for a patient precluded this, then the patients stayed in their own wards or were escorted as appropriate. <u>The whole clinical team came to accept</u> that the <u>granting of leave referred to an arrangement whereby the patient would leave the establishment and sleep out for often days, or even weeks, at a time usually as part of a process of rehabilitation</u>. Within a District General Hospital site the situation is very different. The Psychiatric Unit <u>does not include a cafeteria or shop facilities and patients have to go to other parts of the busy District General Hospital site to access such services</u>. In addition, the hospital is well within walking distance of the town centre and liberally serviced with buses. In retrospect, different constraints are immediately imposed upon the granting of leave but these do not seem to have been thought through.

The procedure adopted at EMC was then explained:

All decisions to grant leave were made by qualified nursing staff. Such decisions would either be made by the key worker or by the person in charge of the team (if not the key worker) in conjunction with the co-worker on duty. Medical staff would be consulted where this was felt to be appropriate. However, where as part of the overall care plan an increasing amount of freedom was implied (e.g. preliminary plans for discharge were being made) separate consent was not sought. All staff are now clear that such practice is outside the requirements of the Act.

The Trust expressed its regrets that the process failed to highlight that 'requests for minor degrees of leave were not being authorised by the RMO and that it had become custom and practice for nurses to assume delegated authority'. It was further acknowledged that no specific documentation was raised in the cases of detained patients' leave of absence; records would appear, as it was claimed, in the nursing notes or in the clinical notes whenever the RMO 'had been *consulted*' (italics supplied).

At the oral hearing on 22 September 1994, Dr John Lambourn (supported by Mrs Pamela Smith and Mr Bill Warr) explained that he and his colleagues, who had come from Exminster Hospital in 1986 carrying their previous practice, considered that the word 'leave' constituted 'absence from the hospital premises for a substantial period of time, usually involving at least a night away from the unit, or at a substantial distance'. He thought that such a definition had 'evolved long before the new Mental Health Act'. That would have been a plausible explanation, were it not for the fact that section 17 of the 1983 Act was a repeat of section 39 of the Mental Health Act 1959 (subject to one slight amendment in section 17(3) which provided for the absentee patient remaining in custody for the purposes of re-arrest if the patient failed to return). The truth of the matter is that the practitioners in mental health in South Devon were in glorious uncertainty about their legal powers and duties. Mr Warr said that during the period of his training in mental health law he had 'never heard of section 17 and I checked that out with recently qualified staff. They all knew section 5(2), sections, 2, 3, 37 and 41 and the more common ones but not many people knew section 17'. The 'more common' sections relate specifically to the legal authority to detain a mentally disordered person. Unlike section 17, they do not deal with the care and treatment of detained patients.

Training in mental health law appears, astonishingly, not to have been part of any curriculum ordained by the Royal College of Psychiatrists. But that unhappy state of affairs is being rapidly repaired. It is essential that anyone in the mental health system should have had some tuition in the Act and the Code of Practice. Anyone exercising the powers and duties derived from statute must be aware of their nature and extent. It is the primary task of management to ensure that practitioners are adequately versed in the law and practice in mental health and, further, that policies and procedure are properly formulated to instruct and guide all practitioners. In the absence of any direct application of the law relating to leave of absence, we examined how in practice the staff at EMC handled the frequent desire of detained patients to move freely in and out of EMC.

In the late 1980s the local coroner, Mr Hamish Turner, expressed his misgivings about the appropriateness of management's response to those patients at EMC who appeared to have been given leave of absence or discharged into the community without sufficient regard to the risk of suicide. A confidential report in November 1989 by Professor H.G. Morgan, professor of psychiatry at the University of Bristol, concluded that the experience in Torbay was not significantly out of line with the national picture. He went on to urge the need for an agreed policy regarding the assessment of the management of suicide risks. He produced a set of guidelines, 'Persons at risk of suicide: guidelines on good clinical practice', January 1990, commending their adoption by the South Devon Healthcare Trust. This was done. What appears to have been overlooked was the proper application of the law relating to the grant of leave of absence, as laid down in section 17, Mental Health Act 1983. The guidelines dealt only with the case of a suicide-risk patient who leaves the ward without notice. An allusion to 'home visits' did no more than stress their health-care value. The possible tragic consequences of an inattention to section 17 leave can be well illustrated by the case of Stephen Hext.

Stephen Hext

Stephen Hext was born on 21 July 1972 and was, by all accounts, a good student with a bright future. In his late teens he exhibited 'symptoms of lack of thought-control and paranoia'. He was first admitted to EMC in November 1992 for assessment under section 2, Mental Health Act 1983. He was compulsorily admitted for treatment in January 1993, remaining a detained patient until mid-March 1993. He had a short spell of six days in EMC in June

1993. His final admission was on 21 November 1993 as an informal patient, which was converted into a compulsory admission on 23 November 1993. Throughout the earlier period of 1993 he was frequently home on leave, some of these occasions during a period of detention and requiring leave from his RMO. (On those occasions leave appeared to be given, in accordance with a long-standing practice, by nursing staff.)

Stephen Hext was allowed out for the day, on 11 December 1993, his first since his admission. That absence was with the permission of nursing staff, and was recorded in the nursing notes. It both followed and succeeded the bi-weekly ward rounds made by Stephen Hext's RMO, Dr Stuart McLaren. While Dr McLaren had unimpeded access to nursing notes, it had never been his practice to read them. He relied instead on being informed orally by nursing staff at his weekly ward rounds of the salient features of the patients' care. Stephen Hext returned from that day's leave, without incident and on time.

On 15 December 1993, at around ten o'clock in the morning, a nursing assistant referred a request from Stephen Hext to leave EMC for the day, to a staff nurse who was the patient's key worker. Leave was granted on condition of a 5 pm return. The key worker said that he regularly made decisions about a patient's mental condition and fitness to go on leave. It was, indeed, common practice for key workers to decide on unrestricted patient's leave. The grant of leave to Stephen Hext on 15 December 1993 was otherwise unconditional. No question of an escort seemed to have been considered. He left EMC and went into Torquay, where he fell to his death from the roof of a multi-storey car park.

At an internal inquiry into the circumstances leading up to the death of Stephen Hext, Bill Warr was asked about the practice of giving leave of absence. (He had not himself been on duty on 15 December 1993.) He is recorded in the inquiry report as stating the following:

> Mr Warr confirmed that it was normal practice for nursing staff to allow patients to leave when under section if felt appropriate and that the doctors were fully aware of this practice. He stated that he himself had attended case reviews when doctors had been informed that a patient under section had been out and, while medical and nursing opinion might be different, the rule was not brought into question.
>
> He stated that when he was a charge nurse working on the Edith Morgan Centre on a number of occasions he informed doctors that

section patients had been out after the event; he was unaware of any discussion about the difference in the rules and the actual practice. When doctors did their ward rounds, if they thought that a patient should be on certain levels of observation, this should be recorded in the nursing notes. He also stated that there was no requirement for nurses to look at medical notes before letting patients out, since it was assumed that all relevant information was in both sets of notes. He also stated that at ward round the doctor in attendance would be told whether any patient had been given leave of absence on an earlier occasion.

The internal inquiry procedure

The Director of Nursing and Patient Services, Mrs Hilary Cunliffe, wrote on 17 January 1994 to Mr Robin Foster, the Assistant Director (Patient Services), asking if he would chair an inquiry, together with Dr Iain MacLeod, the clinical director, and Mrs Carole Heatly, the business manager, into the case of Stephen Hext. The inquiry team – referred to by the team as the 'review panel' – held interviews with three members of nursing staff on 14 February 1994 and a further four members on 30 March 1994. They also interviewed Dr Stuart McLaren. The delay of six weeks between interview dates was said to be 'unavoidable', as a member of the panel was indisposed and it was felt in the best interests of staff that continuity should be maintained throughout. In fact, all the nursing staff were interviewed only by Mr Foster and Mrs Heatly. Dr MacLeod appeared to have 'invited' his two colleagues on the inquiry team to undertake the interviews of the staff members 'on his behalf'. The interview of Dr McLaren was conducted only by Mrs Heatly and Dr MacLeod. The report was submitted to Mrs Cunliffe on 14 April 1994, four months after Stephen Hext's death.

We think this delay in investigating the circumstances of a suicide of a patient in the circumstances outlined above is unacceptable. The NHS Executive (HSG(94)27 of 10 May 1994) has issued guidelines which in part relate to necessary action 'if things go wrong' in managing mentally disordered patients. We think that it is helpful if we recite the guidance given:

> 33. If a violent incident occurs, it is important not only to respond to the immediate needs of the patient and others involved, but in serious cases also to learn lessons for the future. In this event, action by local management must include:

– an immediate investigation to identify and rectify possible short-comings in operational procedures, with particular reference to the Care Programme Approach. Where court proceedings in relation to the incident have started or are thought likely, legal advice should be sought with a view to ensuring that the investigation does not prejudice those proceedings;

– if the victim was a child, ie under 18 years of age, the report of the investigation should be forwarded to the Area Child Protection Committee within one month of the incident.

– incidents involving a death should be reported to the Confidential Inquiry into Homicides and Suicides by Mentally Ill People (telephone 071 823 1031; fax 071 823 1035).

34. Additionally, after the completion of any legal proceedings it may be necessary to hold an independent inquiry. *In cases of homicide, it will always be necessary to hold an inquiry which is independent of the providers involved.* The only exception is where the victim is a child and it is considered that the report by the Area Protection Committee (*see paragraph 33*) fully covers the remit of an independent inquiry as set out below.

35. In cases of suicide of mentally ill people in contact with the specialist mental health services, there must be a local multi-disciplinary audit as specified in *Health of the Nation*.

36. In setting up an independent inquiry the following points should be taken into account:

i. *the remit of the inquiry* should encompass at least:

– the care the patient was receiving at the time of the incident;

– the suitability of that care in view of the patient's history and assessed health and social care needs;

– the extent to which that care corresponded with statutory obligations, relevant guidance from the Department of Health, and local operational policies;

– the exercise of professional judgment

– the adequacy of the care plan and its monitoring by the key worker.

ii. *composition of the inquiry panel*. Consideration should be given to appointing a lawyer as chairman. Other members should include a psychiatrist and a senior social services manager and/or senior nurse. No member of the panel should be employed by bodies responsible for the care of the patient;

iii. *distribution of the inquiry report.* Although it will not always be desirable for the final report to be made public, an undertaking should be given at the start of the inquiry that its main findings will be made available to interested parties.

It is essential that investigation of the death of a patient should always be conducted with expedition. The delay of a month in ordering the inquiry was itself unduly protracted, if not inordinate. Even if the imminence of the Christmas holidays would have made it difficult to convene the team and start the interviews, there is no excuse for management having waited a month. The setting up of the inquiry should have been instantaneous, with the composition of the team perhaps following a few days later, so the interviews could have taken place sooner. A report should have been in the hands of management, at the most within six weeks, and not sixteen. Once the report had been seen and, where necessary, acted upon by management, there is every reason why Stephen Hext's parents should have been supplied with a copy of the report and its recommendations.

It is undesirable that, at the interviews of staff and others, any member of an inquiry team should be absent. Exceptionally, it may be unavoidable that one member of a three-member panel is not present. We think it unfortunate, however, that Dr MacLeod allowed his two colleagues to do all the interviewing, save that of Dr McLaren. And on that occasion only two out of the three sat.

There is obviously a logistical problem of organising the interviewing of individuals consistent with orderliness and speed. But we suggest that an inquiry team might do better to start by instantly collating the documentary evidence – clinical notes and nursing notes. Sometimes it will be helpful to ask potential witnesses to submit a written statement of their involvement in the event under inquiry before interviewing them. Time is a precious commodity. Both time and effort can be economised on if the administrators set out a model procedure to be adopted by inquiry teams, the membership of which may well be clinicians and staff who are not regularly involved in the formal processes of investigation of untoward incidents.

The findings of the internal inquiry

The main issues addressed by the inquiry team were:

1. The policies and procedure relating to leave of absence for unrestricted detained patients.
2. The granting of leave to Stephen Hext to absent himself from the Edith Morgan Centre on 15 December 1993.
3. The awareness of staff of the Code of Practice and the training in its use.
4. The procedure for tracing patients absent without leave.
5. The lack of integration of clinical and nursing notes.

The inquiry team's main concern was the question of the level of communication between nursing and medical staff. It noted that neither read each other's notes, and recommended that both sets of notes should be read and discussed at ward rounds, with the key worker of each patient respectively in attendance. In a later recommendation the inquiry team said that nursing and medical notes should be amalgamated, thus avoiding in the future any separateness flowing from their source. The inquiry team gave priority to this issue, presumably because this practice of separateness of notes directly led to the granting to Stephen Hext of the leave of absence. Dr McLaren stated categorically that he would not himself have granted leave to Stephen Hext, and had he known of the earlier leave of absence (discernible on reading the nursing notes but apparently not alluded to on the ward round) he would have instructed the nursing staff not to permit Stephen Hext to leave EMC. Dr McLaren did not read nursing notes but relied on being told any significant events during his ward round. Dr McLaren was questioned directly on this point by us. We reproduce the questions (from Mr Thorold) and answers:

Q. At the time that you had responsibility for Andrew Robinson, 9th June – 1st September, did you in fact read the nursing notes on Andrew Robinson at all during that time?
A. I didn't, no.
Q. Can you just help to explain why, because in terms of volume, they are not all that considerable to read. On a ward round I presume they were available?
A. They are available but I rely upon a member of the nursing staff

to update myself on the ward round on any developments in behaviour and it is they that use their notes.

Q. Do you still follow that practice?

A. Yes, I do.

Q. So you don't read the nursing notes?

A. On the whole, no.

Q. So if there is information in a nursing note indicating that he has left the Unit with some purported leave, but not in a medical note, you fail to become aware that he is receiving leaves of absence that should not have been granted?

A. That would be one potential way of missing that, yes.

Q. Isn't it simpler for a doctor simply to read the nursing notes, rather than rely on the nursing staff? After all, between let's say the five or seven days between ward rounds it would only take half a minute to read the relevant nursing notes?

A. The way that the ward round is constituted I think that certainly the nursing staff would be unhappy if I talked with them and then read their notes. That is the reason for having a nurse within the ward round.

Q. Would they be less unhappy if you read the notes first and then talked to them?

A. I haven't discussed this formally with the nursing staff.

We trust that such an attitude will not survive the decision that all notes, medical and nursing, should be amalgamated.

The inquiry team stated that 'there has clearly been a liberal interpretation of the Code of Practice and lack of policies and procedures for the Edith Morgan Centre'. This limp finding fails to have regard specifically to the law, and omits placing the responsibility on management for ensuring compliance.

The inquiry team's resort to the Code of Practice as the primary source led to a misapplication of the statutory obligation in section 17, Mental Health Act 1983 which prescribes the granting of leave of absence as being exclusively exercisable by the unrestricted patient's RMO. The statutory provision does not permit a flexible interpretation of the Code which is only guidance as to how the law should be applied. The inquiry team's reliance on the Code as permitting flexibility in the grant of leave of absence is all the more surprising, since on the occasion of the visit to EMC by the Mental Health Act Commission on 24/25 February 1994, the Commissioners specifically raised the need of the Trust to take account of the law, as laid down in section 17 of the Act, and the Code of Practice. The preparation of a policy document by management was pointed up as a glaring omission. On 22 June 1994 the Chairman of the

Psychiatric Consultants Committee wrote to management stating 'that we have now a fully agreed policy covering leave of absence'.

The absence hitherto of any policy and procedure document permitted the nursing staff, as day-to-day carers of patients, to think that they were entitled, at their discretion, to exercise the power, supposedly delegated to them by the consultant psychiatrists. The inquiry team concluded that 'qualified nursing staff were fully aware of the Code of Practice but have to date received no training in it. They also believe that the consultant psychiatrists have devolved the decision-making process of whether a sectioned patient could leave the unit or not to them. Each and every one of them has been making this judgment for some considerable time with, it is said, the full knowledge of the consultant medical staff.' The inquiry team did not ask the consultant psychiatrists as a body about their understanding of the matter. Dr McLaren, Stephen Hext's RMO, told us that he was unaware of a practice which allowed patients leave of absence without the permission of the unrestricted patients' RMO. He was quite adamant – a statement repeated before us at the oral hearings – that only an RMO could grant a detained patient leave of absence; in the case of a restricted patient, only with the express approval of the Home Secretary.

We find it barely credible that the consultant psychiatrists were unaware of the common and long-standing practice of leave of absence being granted by qualified nursing staff. The inquiry team failed to determine whether the assertion of unawareness of the practice has been made good. And we have now conducted our own investigation. In the final analysis we have proceeded upon the assumption that the left hand of medicine did not know what the right hand of nursing was doing – hardly a symbiotic relationship!

The inquiry team declined to recommend any disciplinary action, since the action of the nursing staff in granting leave of absence was in conformity with established practice whereby the consultant psychiatrists (based on the sole evidence of Dr McLaren) had been unaware that leave of absence was being regularly given by nursing staff without direct reference to and approval by the relevant RMO. Dr McLaren was clear about the exclusive authority of the RMO in the granting or refusing of leave of absence.

The fact that such a lack of mutual understanding over the important question of a detained patient's right to be away from the hospital should exist is, we think, a failure primarily attributable to management, contributed to by the absence of effective professional leadership.

ANNEX[2]

20 Leave of Absence (section 17)

20.1 Leave of absence can only be authorized in accordance with the provisions of section 17. It can be an important part of a patient's treatment plan. It is important to note that only the patient's RMO (with the approval of the Home Secretary in the case of a restricted patient) can grant a detained patient leave of absence. The granting of leave should not be used as an alternative to discharging the patient.

20.2 The patient should be fully involved in the decision to grant leave and must be asked to consent to any consultation with others (i.e. relative, professionals in the community) thought necessary before leave is granted. He should be able to demonstrate to his professional carers that he is likely to cope outside the hospital.

20.3 Leave of absence should be well planned (if possible well in advance) and involve detailed consultation with any appropriate relatives/friends (especially where the patient is to reside with them) and community services which could contribute to its successful implementation. If relatives/friends are to be involved in the patient's care, but he does not consent to their being consulted, leave should not be granted. It should be remembered that the duty to provide aftercare (section 117) applies to patients on leave of absence.

20.4 The Power to grant leave (section 17)

a. Unrestricted patients

(i) The decision (which cannot be delegated to another professional) rests with the patient's RMO after necessary consultation (it is not a decision that can be devolved to another doctor), who may impose such condition as he considers necessary. The RMO and other professionals involved should bear in mind, however, that their responsibilities for the patient's care remain the same while he is on leave although they are exercised in a different way. Similarly the aftercare provisions of section 117 apply to a patient on leave of absence;

[2] The underlining indicates the amendments made in the second edition of the Code.

(ii) it is common practice for the RMO, after multi-disciplinary discussions, to authorise short-term local escorted leave at the discretion of nursing staff. Whilst flexibility to respond to day to day changes in a patient's condition is helpful in rehabilitation, there is no formal authority for the RMO to delegate his power under section 17. He must, therefore, accept responsibility for any leave arranged with his general approval;

(iii) where the RMO authorises nurses to arrange discretionary local leave this fact must be recorded. Hospitals should consider the use of a simple record form on which the RMO can authorise leave and specify the conditions attached to it. See para. 20.5.

XVI. Reflections on Practice

There are some things you learn best in calm, and some in storm.*

Providing effective, appropriate and acceptable mental health care is a challenging and complex affair. Severe mental illness does not just affect one segment of the person's life, it affects it all. At the same time,

> having a mental illness, even a severe one, does not suddenly change the basic human search for a full and fulfilling life. Nor does it alter the fundamental requirements on which such a search is necessarily grounded – an appropriate place to live, an adequate income, a meaningful social life, employment or other satisfactory day activity and help and support when in need.[1]

To address the diversity of needs thrown up in the person with severe mental illness is a daunting task for any well-integrated and coordinated team. For any single professional it is well-nigh impossible. The presenting difficulties will be perceived, interpreted and addressed according to the viewpoint, bias and resources of that one professional. The resulting intervention will be, at best, a partial solution. If, on the other hand, several individual professionals are involved, then a selection of interventions may be produced. With luck, these may come together as a complementary patchwork; without coordination, however, the potential for conflicting formulations and interventions is great. The ideal position is achieved when a group of individual professionals come together from their own unique professional perspectives, share their perceptions and formulations, and jointly develop an integrated package of care.

If we look back over Andrew Robinson's history, each of these approaches and the consequences can be clearly seen. While under Dr Conway's care, Andrew was effectively in the hands of a lone practitioner. Other professionals (three successive social workers and one CPN) were involved, but they were marginalised, their

---

* Willa Sibert Cather, *The Song of the Lark* (1915).
[1] *Creating Community Care*, The Mental Health Foundation (1994), p. 17.

overall impact neutralised by Dr Conway's style. Notions of consultation, collaboration, information-sharing and team work were
alien to Dr Conway. Indeed, when asked whether he had had an
opportunity to work in a multi-disciplinary team, Dr Conway told
us: 'I don't think we had teams then. I can't remember. I didn't
think we did.' This comment related to a period from 1983 to 1986.
His diagnosis of Andrew's condition and consequent treatment
were performed entirely independently of those who should have
been regarded as colleagues. Had Dr Conway been amenable to the
contribution of others, events might have unfolded in a very different way.

Andrew's final admission to EMC in June 1993 is a similarly
graphic example of the inadequacies of multi-professional involvement so long as the individuals concerned continued to act
as independent practitioners. Although the various team members met together on a regular basis, there was little evidence
that there was any real sharing of formulation or planning, or of
information about what was happening in the various domains.
The most striking example of this relates to the issue of leave.
If it is true that Dr McLaren was unaware at any time that
Andrew was leaving the unit, let alone on the regular basis that
he was, then that is a very telling indictment of the communication between nursing and medicine. This was not information
that was being withheld; it was being recorded openly, if erratically, in the nursing notes, and any discussion of the detail of
Andrew's daily life would have brought it to light. If this did not
happen, it suggests that the medical gaze was fixed on psycho-
pharmacological issues and formal mental state assessment,
while day-to-day management, social functioning and the activities of daily living were viewed as the domain of nursing – a case
of psychiatric apartheid. No adequate risk-assessment and care
package development could take place against that background.
It was a recipe for tragedy.

This becomes all the more poignant, when considered against
the previous successful episode of care, where, through tight and
well coordinated multi-disciplinary team work, Andrew had been
provided with a framework which had helped him to maintain a
quality of life that had been eluding him since he first came off
medication in 1985. This was the period of Guardianship, which
ran from November 1989 to July 1992. One of the striking features
of the arrangements that were made when the Guardianship Order

was commenced was the detail of the contract that was drawn up between Andrew and the care team. The contract was the result of detailed multi-disciplinary and multi-agency discussions. It set out clearly what was expected of Andrew, and what he could expect and from whom. It addressed a range of aspects of Andrew's life, including accommodation, social contact, meals, self-care and medication. It reflected a rounded vision of Andrew. There were times when Andrew experienced difficulties during this period, but the team was so well-integrated around him that those difficulties could be readily absorbed and addressed in a timely and effective way. It is possible that the success of this period was due solely to the mere existence of the Guardianship Order. It is likely, however, that the key ingredient was the tightly integrated teamwork within the legal constraint of the Order, however limited in its coerciveness. Regrettably, the Guardianship Order was lifted at the same time as the team began to disband, and so whichever had been the dominant factor, the benefit was lost.

These three examples of different styles of professional working, drawn from Andrew's history, are illuminating. The individual practitioner is prone to catastrophic errors of judgement; the collection of professionals who do not communicate effectively are ill-equipped to design comprehensive care packages, simply because no one professional sees the whole picture. The well-integrated team can, on the contrary, design, implement and monitor an effective package, addressing a wide range of needs. Given the discovery of the efficacy of such an approach, it is infinitely regrettable that it was abandoned.

While we fully endorse multi-disciplinary working as the approach of choice, some cautionary notes need to be sounded. Joining with other disciplines in a common endeavour should not mean that professionals abandon their discipline for a generic soup. The nurse holds on to nursing skills and works within a nursing code of conduct; likewise the occupational therapist, the psychologist, the social worker, the doctor, and whoever else may be a member of the team. It is upon a firm base of understanding of the individual professional skills, competencies and responsibilities that true collaboration can be built. The role of the RMO in this context, vis-à-vis his legal powers to grant leave of absence, provides an appropriate commentary.

There is no provision within this section of the Act for leave to be granted by anyone other than the patient's RMO, in conjunction with the Home Office in the case of restricted patients. This is not a duty that can be delegated. Circumstances in which leave is granted by nursing staff unbeknown to the RMO, are, therefore, patently unlawful.

As the law currently stands, the RMO is under no obligation to consult with any other party when granting leave. There is, of course, nothing to prevent him from consulting colleagues, so long as he retains the exclusive power to grant or refuse leave. We believe that consultation accords with the principles of multi-disciplinary working, discussed above. A model of good practice in relation to section 17 leave would require that the timing of, the criteria for, and the conditions surrounding the granting of leave would be included as an integral part of the multi-disciplinary care planning process. A protocol for granting leave would be drawn up for each patient and, wherever possible, with the full involvement of the patient. The RMO has the ultimate responsibility for the detail contained within that protocol. Once agreed and in place, the protocol could be actioned by any designated member of the multi-disciplinary team. The RMO would be informed of each period of leave as granted and the conditions of leave would be subject to review at intervals agreed within the protocol. The protocol would include details of the type of leave to be granted – escorted or unescorted; and, if escorted, by whom. It would also include the limits on the duration and the frequency of the leave, the earliest start date, any contraindications that would disqualify the patient from leave and any sanctions to be applied if there has been non-compliance with the terms and conditions for leave. It would list by name and office those people to whom the authority to grant leave within the terms of the protocol might be delegated. Such a development would, we believe, ensure that the principles behind the current section 17 were upheld, while enabling the application to be updated in line with current practice. We do not think that such a procedure requires an amendment to section 17. But clearly it should be spelt out in a third edition of the Code of Practice. So long as the RMO continues to exercise the power exclusively, others may properly execute that power.

A thorough and correct understanding of the roles and responsibilities of each member of the team is essential for effective multi-disciplinary working. Another essential component is high quality communication. A review of Andrew Robinson's history reveals countless examples of ineffective communication. Despite the importance that is attached to discharge summaries, there was scarcely one that did not include either factual inaccuracies or distortions, or both. A prime example of the genre is Dr Cullen's summary of November 1986, but this is not a lone example. If discharge summaries are to be regarded as credible sources of information – and there is little point to them unless they can be so regarded – then they must be accurate, not only in their record of the immediate episode of care, but also in their outline of the patient's historical perspective. No finer model can be cited than Dr Exworthy's summary, which forms Appendix 2 to this report.

While there is a responsibility on discharging carers to provide full and accurate information, there is also a responsibility on receiving carers to ensure that they are in possession of all relevant material. Throughout his post-Broadmoor care, little attempt was made by any professional to obtain source material about Andrew's index offence. Most professionals had an understanding that there had been a firearm involved, but the nature of that involvement varied considerably. In his undated report to the MHRT in 1986 Dr Conway wrote: 'While at this University, he formed a romantic liaison with a woman some six years his senior and when this relationship broke up, he is alleged to have gone to her room with a shot gun.' Although he initially dismissed the distinction as 'splitting hairs', Dr Conway did acknowledge to us that – apart from using the dismissive word 'alleged' – there was a difference between thinking that Andrew had just wanted to frighten his girlfriend with a gun, as he had understood to be the case, and hearing that he had wanted to maim her with the shotgun, as described in Andrew's statement to the police.

Dr Conway was not alone in under-playing the risk that Andrew presented. Repeatedly, the more threatening aspects of Andrew's behaviour were minimised, and the violence in his ideation was not taken on board by clinicians working with him. Through the course of the Inquiry, again and again it seemed that otherwise skilled clinicians were blinded to the potential risk that Andrew posed by his charm, his intelligence, or by his ability to mask his symptoms, at least for short periods. Those attributes may have accounted for why information that was available had failed to register, while information that was not readily to hand was not sought. Without all available information, accurate risk-assessment becomes impossible. We would, therefore, urge that an index of essential documentation is developed to serve as a check list for newly-referred patients. This should form the basis of a minimum documentation standard, at least in relation to patients with a forensic background, or on supervision (or mental health priority) registers.

So far, we have assessed the issue of sequential recording. It would be a mistake to assume that there are no problems with concurrent information-sharing. We have already alluded to the situation pertaining in EMC between June and August 1993. According to Dr McLaren, he was completely unaware that Andrew was having periods of leave outside the unit. To the nursing staff, absences with leave were common knowledge and they were spasmodically recorded in the nursing notes. These notes were freely available to all disciplines, and were regularly consulted by the junior doctors. One step that could and should have been taken as a matter of urgency, was the abandonment of separate professional notes, and the development of multi-disciplinary records. At the same time as integrating professional notes into a single record, attention should be paid to integrating hospital and community records. The ideal to aim for is a single mental health record for each patient, irrespective of where they are treated, or by whom. On its own, this will not resolve the blockage around information-sharing, but it will remove an unnecessary hurdle. Coupled with the development of a genuinely multi-disciplinary team approach, improvement should be marked.

A further consideration in improving practice is the role of supervision. Supervision is 'an intensive, interpersonally focused, one-to-one relationship in which one person is designated to facilitate the development of competence in the other person'.[2]

This is one definition, of which there are many variants. The basic premise remains constant. Even the most skilled and experienced amongst us can benefit from reflecting on our practice under the guidance of a skilled practitioner whom we trust. Within social work and psychotherapy, this is a well established practice. For nursing, it has long been a feature of community work. It is rapidly gaining ground in other settings. *Working in Partnership*[3] recommends 'that new training initiatives aimed at developing clinical supervision skills in senior clinical nurses are devised. We also recommend that newly qualified nurses and nursing students receive preparation in what to expect from clinical supervision'.

[2] Hawkins and Shohet, *Supervision in the Helping Professions* (1988) OUP.
[3] *Working in Partnership* (1994) HMSO, London.

We would fully support that recommendation, and would further support the extension of the principle to all mental health professionals at all grades. It became evident during the Inquiry that, although there was a measure of supportive supervision for junior doctors as part of their training, at consultant level no such provision was available. This reflects the national picture. Even when such lack of supervision does not result in flawed clinical judgment, the additional burden that it places upon consultants is unsustainable in the long term.

At this juncture, comment must be passed on the arrangements for nursing supervision in South Devon. From January 1993 Bill Warr had the dual role of Nurse Advisor (Mental Health) and Manager for EMC. On both counts he had a responsibility to ensure that effective systems were in place to provide the nursing staff with appropriate supervision. Mr Warr acknowledged that such systems were not in place during 1993, although that deficit is now being urgently addressed. Of rather more concern to us is the absence of supervision available to Mr Camus who, as an Enrolled Nurse, was, during the period of Andrew's last community relapse, carrying a burden of responsibility far beyond that which was appropriate for his grade. There was a systems failure that allowed such a situation to develop and then go unchallenged. There was an individual failure on the part of the Nurse Advisor for failing to establish an effective system. Our criticism of Mr Warr in that respect has to be viewed against the impossible burden of dual posts imposed on him by top management. It is a matter of mitigation.

This leads onto consideration of the general context within South Devon Health Care Trust that enabled some of the issues outlined above to gain a foothold. This is not the place to reiterate the findings of our earlier review of the mental health services. Suffice it to say, we have found nothing during this Inquiry that has made us reconsider the views expressed in our first report. The flaws in the system, particularly around senior management and professional leadership, had a direct bearing on the care and treatment of Andrew Robinson and, therefore, contributed to the death of Georgina Robinson.

XVII. Listening to Supporters

Lord Chief Justice of the King's Bench:
I think you are fallen into the disease [of selective deafness] for you
hear not what I say to you.

Sir John Falstaff:
Very well my Lord, very well: rather, an't please you, it is the disease
of not listening, the malady of not marking, that I am troubled
withal.*

Throughout this inquiry we had ample evidence of the heavy and
distressing burden borne by Andrew Robinson's parents, both
when he was living with them and when they were trying to support
him while he was living nearby, and worrying about him when he
was in hospital. We had the overwhelming impression that, with a
few notable exceptions, the professionals' attitude to the Rev. and
Mrs Robinson was 'semi-detached', that professionals did not regard them as part of the caring team, merely as interested parties
watching from the touchlines but never part of the scrimmage of
mental health services. The services did not attempt to engage
them in the care plans made for their son; their letters to professionals in the service are moving testimony to their recurrent
despair about Andrew's mental illness and unsatisfactory situation
at times of deepening crisis, when the shadow of impending disaster grew longer. The overwhelming impression they gained was
that professionals paid more attention to their own brief interviews
with Andrew than they did to family and friends who were in daily
contact with him; that it was frequently difficult to get access to
see someone quickly or to evoke a prompt response; and that, while
they bore the brunt of caring for their son, they were rarely kept
fully informed of changes in his care plan. After Andrew Robinson's
discharge from Moorhaven Hospital in 1986, for example, Dr Conway having decided that his patient's main problems were due to
a 'personality disorder', the Rev. Peter Robinson recalled, in his
written evidence to us:

* *Henry IV, Part 2*, I.2.136-41.

Clearly the staff at Moorhaven did not realise how ill he was, but as soon as he was released and came home, at the beginning of October 1986, it was immediately apparent, not only to us but to all our neighbours and those who visited the house, that he was very ill indeed. He demanded to be sent abroad to escape 'the Nazi dictatorship in this country' and he seemed to be in a constant state of fear, locking and bolting doors and making sure the curtains were tightly drawn, and he complained of being radiated by nuclear rays which he said were being directed at him from Devonport dockyard via the television or radio. If we switched on either he became very disturbed. The Chernobyl disaster triggered this off. He kept telephoning people all over the country, including the Prime Minister at 10 Downing Street, and when I put a lock on the instrument he broke it. Sometimes he would pace up and down in a very agitated state, at other times he would wander outside without any shoes and stand motionless in the rain for long periods of time, and once he sat slumped on the bathroom floor for several hours in a catatonic state. He would cry out in terror because he thought flames were coming through the floorboards or he was being shot at through the window. Afterwards he seemed to have no recollection of these events. As we did not seem to be getting any response from the authorities I finally wrote to our MP.

... his behaviour had become increasingly violent, and he was particularly angry with us for not sending him abroad. At nights we had to lock our bedroom door to get some sleep. A copy of a letter my wife wrote to MIND gives some idea of the state of despair to which we were reduced.

Referring again to the period when his son was under Dr Conway's care, the Rev. Peter Robinson told us:

It was early in 1985 that medication was stopped. We were not informed of this and Andrew told us nothing but within a few weeks we began to notice a change in attitude. We arranged an interview with Dr Conway on one or two occasions but unfortunately Andrew was invited to be present and it was impossible to voice our concerns.

Referring to Andrew's supervision in the community while he was under a Guardianship Order between 1989 and 1992, the Rev. Peter Robinson wrote:

We were always a little uncertain as to who was in overall charge of him. At first we assumed it was the consultant psychiatrist, but this was not apparently the case, and it was difficult to work out who was ultimately responsible for him.

We should make it clear that during the Guardianship years members of the clinical team did take account of Andrew Robinson's parents' views, were willing to see them and discuss Andrew's case, although not always with the alacrity or the kind of response one might have wished for.

During the early months of 1993, while the professionals negotiated who was to take over responsibility for care, the Robinsons tried again, unsuccessfully, to get professionals to understand the deteriorating situation. Mrs Robinson phoned John Camus many times – he visited, but made his own, independent assessment of the situation. Andrew Robinson was able to behave quite normally for short periods of time and hence able, for the duration of a brief visit, to hide his psychotic experiences from professionals. On 8 March 1993, the Rev. Peter Robinson wrote to John Camus:

> I am sure you are aware that, since ceasing to take medication last November, Andrew has become very unwell, and, as always when he refuses medication, we know (from 16 years experience!) that it can only end in some disaster. We feel as though we are sitting waiting for a time-bomb to go off!

Mr Camus visited Andrew on 9 March but was refused entry. After further phone calls from Mrs Robinson, Dr Monteiro visited on 12 March, but the clinical note made by John Camus of his assessment remarked: 'Although psychotic, he was not as "sick" as we had been led to believe.' The professionals evidently did not think that a time-bomb was ticking away; in that they were over-reliant on a snap-shot opinion which Andrew was adept at evoking.

As negotiations between the teams about Andrew's future care proceeded over the next few months, his parents witnessed a frightening deterioration. In a letter of some desperation, Mrs Robinson wrote to the Director of Social Services, Devon County Council, on May 14 1993:

> I am writing with the gravest concern in connection with our son, Andrew, who suffers from schizophrenia.
>
> When anyone sees Andrew for a short while he presents normally, but most of the time he spends lying on his bed and is gripped by a jumble of thoughts going through his head which he puts down on paper sending masses of illegible and incomprehensible letters to everyone he knows (without stamps).
>
> He was seen walking in the middle of the road in Torquay a few days ago. He is unable to care for himself and for the past 3 months

I have been going to his flat to wash and clean and take prepared food. (The landlord, at Andrew's request, disconnected the stove as he nearly set fire to the flat.) He just sits in the dark if the electricity meter runs out and says 'I am not allowed to have any light'.

As parents we are deeply distressed and with his past history feel this can only end in tragedy if he continues to go without medication.

The wheels of the mental health services turned slowly in response to this letter, although, to his credit, Dr McLaren had responded promptly to an earlier letter from Mr and Mrs Robinson, by inviting them to come and see him to discuss Andrew. Another month of deepening psychosis passed before Andrew Robinson was admitted to hospital.

If close relatives, including Andrew's next of kin, had difficulty in getting their voices heard, then it is perhaps not surprising that other friends and supporters had even greater difficulty in generating a response to their cries for help. Mrs Marian Ingram, a friend of Mrs Robinson, whose acquaintance had been renewed at a carers' meeting, agreed to visit Andrew through the winter of 1992/93 while he was staying in his parents' home in Sidmouth during their absence on holiday in South Africa. Mrs Ingram understood from Mrs Robinson that Andrew would be going every three weeks to Torquay for his injection and would be monitored by Mr Camus. Mrs Ingram's role was to 'keep an eye on him, to do a bit of washing and a few chores'. Mrs Ingram kept a diary between November 1992 and February 1993, a detailed weekly account of Andrew's increasingly worrying condition, revealing her attempts to get help. In her letter to the Inquiry, Mrs Ingram wrote:

During the time that I was visiting and doing things for Andrew, although I made numerous requests from people whom I thought would be concerned, there seemed no one who could do anything constructive to help Andrew, particularly with regard to him having his medication. I felt helpless and frustrated and for some time had wondered what the outcome might be.

I do not need to say that if someone could have done something at the time I was crying out for help for Andrew, this unfortunate incident would not have taken place.

and in a letter of 19 April 1993 to Neil Lindup, MIND development worker, she described her experiences visiting Andrew Robinson:

I made discreet enquiries about injections and discovered that these were not being asked for or given. During the next couple of months

I noticed the deterioration of this man's mental health; he was utterly confused and imagining all sorts of things. Each time I came away I wondered what I would find on my return the following week. I rang the Rehab Centre expressing my concern but was told there was little they could do if he refused to have his injections. They seemed to think it was an imposition my ringing them. I got the same answer from all the various authorities and felt like knocking my head against a brick wall. I was so concerned for him because his parents were out of the country and yet no one seemed to care. Unless something really serious happened, no action could be taken.

Mr Lindup, an experienced voluntary organisation worker, now a manager at MIND in Exeter, had a not dissimilar experience. He wrote to us:

From Christmas 1992 onwards however, I noticed a steady deterioration in Andrew's condition (as did Mrs Ingram and Alan Worthington of the NSF, who were both in contact with him). Andrew stopped coming to our Contact Centres and I saw him at home several times, where he was becoming very disturbed and distressed. As a lay person I would describe him as being tormented. He was not looking after himself and living in some squalor. He also started sending us copies of his book, of which some of the content were very disturbing. I rang John Camus at least four times to inform him of his deterioration, and of the book, but I am afraid I did not make entries in my diary to this effect and can give no dates. Mr Camus reassured me that I was not to worry, but I would have liked to have seen more regular visits and I do feel the East Devon team should perhaps have been involved to a greater extent. I did not feel at all threatened by Andrew, but I did feel sorry for him in his mental torment and anguish. I feel perhaps that I should have been told that he had refused his medication, though I had guessed that this was in fact the case.

It is hardly necessary to comment on these telling extracts, save to say that we believe Andrew Robinson's family's and friends' experiences are not unusual. In our earlier review of the South Devon Mental Health Services, many caring relatives recounted similar experiences.

Improving relationships between professionals and patients' relatives

The Trust should develop a clear policy about the values, principles and practices which govern relationships between staff and patients' close relatives, recognising relatives' rights to information, practical assistance and involvement in care and treatment plans; and their need for emotional support and help. We came across examples of good practice in the Trust during this inquiry which, if fostered across the Trust, would substantially alter relatives' ability to be effective carers and perhaps in part relieve the burden they experience.

More time should be set aside for discussions with relatives about care and treatment plans, and they should be welcomed at case conferences. Some adult patients may, of course, choose not to accept the involvement of their close family relatives in their care. There will also, on occasions, be matters which have no bearing on the relatives' ability to care for the patient which a patient wishes to remain confidential between him and his doctor or key worker. But, in those very common circumstances where the patient is receiving substantial emotional or practical support from relatives, they surely have a right to know sufficient details about the mental disorder, its likely course, warning symptoms of relapse and how and when to summon help, to enable them to discharge their responsibilities effectively. The key task in working with relatives is to *engage* them in the overall care plan so that they become partners with the clinical team in their relative's care.

The Rev. Peter Robinson made the following recommendation:

Psychiatric and social workers need to take warnings from the *family* that a patient's condition is deteriorating much more seriously than they do at present.

We wholeheartedly endorse that view. Professionals need to be trained to trust the experienced judgment of close family, rather than rely on their own impressions made at one isolated assessment.

Working with friends, neighbours, voluntary agency workers and other supporters

Neil Lindup, when asked for his view about how best professionals might communicate better with voluntary workers (bearing in mind the issue of confidentiality of some information between the patient and his doctors), described to us a very good working relationship he felt he had established with the neighbouring East Devon Mental Health Team:

I have got a very good rapport with the East Devon Mental Health
Team, to be honest. I think that they trust me and I trust them.

When asked to expand on how the relationship worked, Mr Lindup
said:

Partly that the team was involved in the setting up of East Devon
MIND, in fact. Eugene Mullin [East Devon Mental Health Service]
was one of the prime movers in setting up East Devon MIND, and
the Social Services Manager, Richard Murray, was also involved so
we have got, I think, a really good working relationship with both
sides. If I am worried about somebody who comes to the drop-in who
seems to be particularly depressed or distressed or something I do
in fact ring up the team and say 'Look, I am not a professional person
but could you just bear in mind that I wasn't very happy with ... John
or Jean or whatever it was ... when I last saw them', because
probably I am seeing them more often than they are, in fact.
Professor Murphy: You would not be asking them to give you information?
Mr Lindup: No.
Professor Murphy: You would be looking for a listening ear?
Mr Lindup: Yes.
Professor Murphy: A very responsive listening ear?
Mr Lindup: Yes. I would hope that they didn't just consider it was a
lay person and therefore they could dismiss it, but rather it was
somebody who, all right was a lay person, but who had got to know
the people quite well as friends, which is what most of the people
who come to our service are, in fact, and I feel that I do know when
they are not up to much. There may be issues of confidentiality there
which are wrong, in fact, but I err on the side of safety rather than
on holding back and letting something happen which could have
been prevented.

Mr Lindup's approach seems to us to strike just the right note. He
accepted that he would not receive confidential information about
patients from professionals, but would expect to be heard and to
have his concerns taken seriously and, on occasion, would breach,
with proper discretion, a patient's confidences to him in order to
protect the patient or others from harm. Professionals in South
Devon should aspire to develop the same sort of trusting relationship with supporters that seems to have been achieved in East
Devon between MIND and the statutory services.

Listening to the community

It was not only relatives and supporters whose cries for help often went unheard. Mrs A., the victim of Andrew Robinson's delusional obsession in 1988 and 1989, was driven to seek the assistance of a solicitor, Mr John Hansell, to negotiate on her behalf with Dr Moss and other parties to ensure that she was protected from Andrew Robinson. There is an inventory of over 30 letters written by Mr Hansell on her behalf at that time. Looking back, Mr Hansell commented that the tone of the correspondence was 'somewhat more emotive language than I would normally use in writing letters on behalf of clients. I felt the situation was very serious and I had to express myself in the light of that background.' Mr Hansell had great difficulty in acquiring information from the services about Andrew Robinson and also at first in getting the services to take his client's problems seriously. When asked at the oral hearings how he would like to see members of the public, like Mrs A., assisted in putting their concerns across to professionals, Mr Hansell stressed the importance of a personal visit from a member of professional staff, to assess the truth of the allegations and to hear at first hand the facts of the problem. We strongly endorse this approach. The key worker, the responsible CPN or team social worker, would be ideally placed to make such a visit to a member of the public in Mrs A.'s situation. No breach of confidentiality will normally be involved in receiving and assessing information but, if there is a clear risk to a member of the public, then there is an over-riding duty to breach confidence and to provide information in so far as it is necessary in the interests of a potential victim. Members of the public should not have to go to a solicitor for assistance in communicating their fears about someone to the local mental health team, although in this case one should be thankful that Mrs A. had Mr Hansell protecting her interests so persistently and, after much effort, effectively.

XVIII. Admission under the Mental Health Act 1983

> If it is necessary to wait until the signs of disorder were so gross that they would be obvious to a lay magistrate, then it would often be too late to institute effective treatment.*

The verb 'to section', meaning to admit to hospital under compulsion, first appeared in the Concise Oxford English Dictionary in the most recent edition published in 1990. The adjective 'sectionable', derived from it, has not yet been included, but probably soon will be. It is common jargon, well understood by mental health professionals. It appeared in the Inquiry documentation many times. 'Sectionable' means having the quality of mental disorder, in the judgment of professionals, which satisfies the criteria for compulsory admission under the provisions of the Mental Health Act. Put very simply, a person is 'sectionable' when the doctors making the recommendations agree that, in their clinical judgment, the criteria in the Act are satisfied, and when the Approved Social Worker making the application is convinced of the case for compulsory admission.

The threshold level of severity of disorder for making this decision is not defined either by the Act or by any specific guidance in the Code of Practice. The judgment is left to individual professionals, who will, of course, take into account the necessity of being able to defend their judgment to Hospital Managers or a Mental Health Review Tribunal. The threshold of disorder which might trigger compulsion varies from one service to another, between different doctors, between indiviual social workers, and also changes over time, as political and public attitudes shift.

The question whether Andrew Robinson should have, or could have been readmitted to hospital at an earlier stage of his relapsing mental illness came up on several occasions during the course of his illness, between the absolute discharge from all legal powers in September 1986 and his final readmission in June 1993.

We, and our counsel Oliver Thorold, puzzled over the dilemmas

---

* Comment by the Lunacy Commissioners on the lunacy legislation of 1890.

faced by the clinicians. While we set forth arguments below as to why Andrew Robinson could have, and should have been detained more promptly, we bear in mind the climate of opinion within which the clinicians were working in the late 1980s and the early 1990s. We remember, too, that there has been a very significant shift of opinion in the last two years, as a result of well-publicised untoward events involving discharged patients, and as a result of the highlighting of the criteria for compulsory admission in the Revised (1993) Code of Practice for the Mental Health Act.[1]

Most of the doctors who gave oral evidence were asked to describe their personal approach to making a recommendation, and we believe their views accord with the prevailing wisdom among practising psychiatrists. But before mentioning their opinions, we examine first what guidance is available from the Act, the Code, and from other sources.

The criteria in the Act

An application for admission for *assessment* (section 2), for a period not exceeding 28 days, may be made in respect of a patient on the grounds that:

(a) he is suffering from mental disorder of a nature or degree which warrants the detention of the patient in a hospital for assessment (or for assessment followed by medical treatment) for at least a limited period; and

(b) he ought to be so detained in the interests of his own health or safety or with a view to the protection of other persons.

An application for admission for *treatment* (section 3) may be made on the grounds that:

(a) he is suffering from mental illness, severe mental impairment, psychopathic disorder or mental impairment and his mental disorder is of a nature or degree which makes it appropriate for him to receive medical treatment in a hospital; and

(b) in the case of psychopathic disorder or mental impairment, such treatment is likely to alleviate or prevent a deterioration of his condition; and

(c) it is necessary for the health or safety of the patient or for the

---

[1] *Code of Practice for the Mental Health Act 1983.* 2nd ed. (1993) HMSO, London.

protection of other persons that he should receive such treatment and it cannot be provided unless he is detained under this section.

For an admission for treatment under section 3 the doctors must state their reasons why other methods of dealing with the patient are not appropriate. The section requires the detention in hospital to be necessary, a more imperative term than 'ought' in section 2.

The Code of Practice

The Code of Practice lists numerous factors to be taken into account in making a decision to admit compulsorily. Among those factors is (para 2.9) 'any evidence suggesting that the patient's mental health will deteriorate if he does not receive treatment', but the guidance does not directly address the issue of how severely disordered a person must be before the criteria are satisfied.

Case law

The principal legal authority, following the 1983 Act, which has addressed the threshold for compulsory admission was *R* v. *Hallstrom, ex parte W*.[2] In the course of his judgment in that case, Mr Justice McCullough said:

> In my judgment, the key to the construction of s.3 lies in the phrase 'admission for treatment'. It stretches the concept of 'admission for treatment' too far to say that it covers admission for only so long as it is necessary to enable leave of absence to be granted [under s.17] after which the necessary treatment will begin. 'Admission for treatment' under s.3 is intended for those whose condition is believed to require a period of treatment as an inpatient. It may be that such patients will also be thought to require a period of outpatient treatment thereafter, but the concept of 'admission for treatment' has no applicability to those whom it is intended to admit and detain for a purely nominal period, during which no necessary treatment will be given.

It should be noted that Mr Justice McCullough was exposing the illegality of purporting to rely on a clinically functionless admission to hospital, an admission that was really no more than a device. His interpretation sets a very low legal standard for compulsory

[2] [1986] QB 1090d.

admission, but does not address the severity of the disorder in clinical terms. The test is simply whether more than a 'nominal' period of inpatient treatment is required. Provided that professional judgments on the other relevant criteria are made in good faith, and this test is met, the law leaves the rest to professionals.

The 'deteriorating patient'

An issue which has generated much confusion and uncertainty concerns the 'sectionability' of the patient whose mental health is likely to deteriorate. Often this issue comes into sharp focus when a patient defaults on medication. Many psychiatrists have assumed that even though a patient has a life-long continuous predisposition to acute psychotic breakdown, if he is not 'mad' enough, in other words not exhibiting gross symptoms, such as frank delusional ideas or experiencing hallucinations, the criteria for detention cannot be satisfied.

We are reminded of the now-discredited approach of ophthalmologists advising patients to wait for their cataracts to 'ripen' before seeking a lens replacement. In a similar way it seems that often – too often – psychiatrists wait for psychotic symptoms to ripen before resorting to the powers in the Mental Health Act. The belief that the Act does not allow compulsory admission to prevent a relapse has undeniably held a powerful grip on mental health professionals and legal writers alike. At the request of the Secretary of State, the Department of Health set up an Internal Review of legal powers for the care of mentally ill people in the community. In its Report[3] the Review Team wrote:

> The 1983 Act requires a patient to be actually suffering from a mental illness at the time of a diagnosis which is used to support an application for admission or guardianship. The Act is not couched in terms of 'futurity' which would allow a patient to be admitted simply on the grounds that his or her past medical history suggests that he or she will relapse in the future.

Similarly, Richard Jones in his Mental Health Act Manual, commenting on the meaning of 'suffering from' in section 3 writes:

---

[3] *Legal Powers on the Care of Mentally Ill People in the Community*, Report of the Internal Review, Department of Health: August 1993.

An anticipated relapse based on the patient's medical history of mental disorder is not sufficient to meet this criterion.[4]

At the heart of this issue, although it is not the only issue, lies the question of what the Act requires for a person to be said to be 'suffering from mental illness'. We believe that both the Internal Review and Richard Jones are wrong.

The case of *Devon County Council* v. *Hawkins*[5] is, surprisingly, not cited in any of the leading legal textbooks on mental health. Yet it is highly pertinent to the issue. The case involved the question whether a person who was taking drugs which successfully controlled his epilepsy could be said to be 'suffering from' epilepsy for the purpose of determining fitness to hold a driving licence.[6] The then Lord Chief Justice, Lord Parker held:

> It is said, and said with much force, that so long as it is necessary for a person to be under treatment for a disease or disability, then that person must be held to be suffering from that disease or disability. In my judgment that is in general right. The respondent, as it seems to me, was suffering from a condition which no doubt is properly termed a disease, a condition of epilepsy, whereby he was subject to attacks, and, as the facts show, these drugs prevented those attacks, in other words prevent the disease from manifesting itself, and so long as drugs are necessary to prevent the manifestation of disease, the disease in my judgment remains. Of course a time may come when drugs are really unnecessary when it could be said that the man is cured, but here on the evidence it appears that as recently as 1963 manifestations occurred when he on his own initiative had ceased taking the drugs.

This decision has remained unchallenged ever since in its own context of road traffic law. We find the parallels in the nature of mental illness entirely apt and compelling. It surely shows that 'futurity' is integral to the analysis, regardless of whether the verbs in the statutory criteria are couched in the future tense. The court was saying that, *if* Mr Hawkins ceased taking his anticonvulsant medication, *then* he would be likely to suffer further epileptic seizures. What he was 'suffering from' rested on a prognosis of what would occur *in the future* if medication was withdrawn.

In Andrew Robinson's case his liability to relapse whenever medication was stopped was absolutely clear by 1988, if not earlier. When he refused further medication in the final part of 1992, after a period under Guardianship, there was really no doubt that a further relapse would occur. It was just as certain as it would be if anti-convulsants were withdrawn from someone with chronic epilepsy.

The timing of a decision to 'section' is often a delicate matter. We proceed to explore the attitudes and approaches of the principal clinicians involved with Andrew Robinson in the first half of 1993.

The final phase

In his opening to the oral hearings, Mr Thorold took us through the events in early January 1993 when Andrew Robinson's mental state was causing anxiety in the community. Dr Jon Wride, a Community Medical Officer (unusually, a GP working with a community team, in this case the Culverhay Community Team in Paignton), was seeing Andrew at that time. Dr Wride was not approved under section 12 of the Mental Health Act, but had experience in psychiatry as a trainee.

In his statement he said that he was aware in late 1992 that Andrew Robinson was refusing his full depot injection. Dr Moss had finished his employment at Culverhay by this time. Dr Wride arranged to 'bump into' Andrew Robinson on 25 January 1993. He was struck by how well he seemed. The meeting was clearly amicable. Andrew even showed some insight into his condition. He accepted the need to be seen to be under the care of a consultant psychiatrist, and appeared ready to meet his new psychiatrist, Dr Monteiro, three weeks later.

By the time that Dr Wride saw him next, on 18 February 1993, there had been reports from the Sidmouth police that Andrew had been following a boy there. He had failed to keep his appointment with Dr Monteiro two days earlier. Dr Wride went to Andrew's flat in Torquay when he appeared to him more agitated, with a paranoid flavour to the content of his speech; he appeared to have lost the earlier insight. He became angry and accusatory when he was asked about his missed appointment with Dr Monteiro, and demanded that his visitors leave. Dr Wride thought that, in the

absence of psychotic features, it would be difficult to justify compulsory admission, though, not having section 12 approval, he
recognised that the decision would have to be made by others. This
event was relayed to Dr Monteiro, who felt that Andrew should be
given time to 'cool off'.

As on so many previous occasions, once more Andrew Robinson's
father, by now back from South Africa, sounded the alarm. He
wrote to John Camus on 8 March saying that, since ceasing to take
medication, his son was again very unwell, that he feared a disaster, and that it was like 'waiting for a time bomb to go off'.

On 12 March, after some strange letters had been received,
Andrew was seen by Dr Monteiro, who found him 'evidently deteriorating'. Dr Monteiro was aware of a letter sent on 3 March by
Andrew indicating that he was preoccupied with killing again. This
did not produce the resolve to 'section' him. At our oral hearings,
Dr Monteiro stressed that he regarded it as most important that
the patient should display demonstrable evidence of marked disturbance before implementing a 'section'. Referring to Andrew's
self control and general presentation in March 1993, which he felt
prevented him from making a recommendation, he said:

> I had also had the experience of being in Tribunals with people who
> were, I thought, worse than he was presenting, who had got off their
> Section, so I felt that it wasn't appropriate at that time to take that
> route. If I had asked for a Section and it had been refused, I would
> have spoilt any possibility of seeing him at a later time.

> Mr Thorold: Refused by hospital managers or a social worker?

> Dr Monteiro: Well, the chances are that it might have been a social
> worker and if the social worker had refused to Section him based on
> his mental state at that time, he would have been very aware of what
> my wishes were towards him and I would have found it impossible
> to maintain a relationship later.

Even as late as June 1993, when he finally completed a section 4
emergency application, Dr Monteiro was wrestling with his con-
science about the explicitness of the symptoms:

> He was extremely plausible and it was actually quite difficult for me
> to get information from him which was psychotic, but I finally did so
> by being slightly provocative with him, and he then went off into
> some thought disorder material which I felt was enough evidence for
> me to proceed with the Section.

So even in the face of overwhelming evidence from family, friends, CPN key worker, and the police of a deteriorating psychotic state, a psychiatrist believes he must have more, and still more compelling evidence.

Dr Christopher Gillespie, when asked his opinion on the right point to admit under the Mental Health Act, replied:

> Well, with him I think that after he defaulted and stopped taking his medication one would have to consistently up-date that – you know, on a weekly basis, almost. I guess that one would be thinking about Mental Health Act intervention very soon, Within a month, at least – six weeks [of his defaulting].

Dr Gillespie stressed the importance of regular monitoring by a consultant, or an experienced senior registrar, and a senior level nurse, so that the patient could be rapidly readmitted, but emphasised the problem that he felt an application for admission could not be made early on, because 'he was capable of presenting quite well until he deteriorated to the point it was fairly obvious he was ill'.

Dr Moss stressed, as Dr Monteiro did, the importance of maintaining a good relationship with one's own patients, and that this necessarily influenced the point at which one recommended intervention, since it might later be resented by the patient. Thus he was influenced by his, and his team's commitment to supporting Andrew, and the desire to reward his success during the Guardianship period by reducing the medication if possible, by removing the Guardianship Order, and by deciding not to 'section' him again, or replace the order when he defaulted on medication.

> I think that I, and my colleagues, find that situation difficult to exercise in practice, judging when the precise behaviour that is reported, which is often just an indicator and a mild change, has reached the stage where one should go to these extents and risk upsetting the whole relationship with the patient. As I have been commenting about this today, I have put myself back in the situation where I recognise how difficult it is to carry that responsibility from an emotional point of view. There are a number of pressures on the Responsible Medical Officer, and I think that is why I have been leaning to say that I, as a consultant, needed some objective situation in which to look at and rehearse the pros and cons of taking these sorts of actions, because I had been through a period, at the end of the Guardianship Order in this case in 1992, where we had put a lot of effort into achieving the degree of improvement that we had as a

team. I had an emotional investment in that. I was pleased that the team had achieved this. Then to be asked almost immediately to become heavy-handed again, and so on, places a great strain. It is part of the task of the RMO, but nevertheless to be aware of the emotional factors at the many levels that are operating in that situation.

These, then, were the responses of the psychiatrists to the question whether, and if so when to invoke compulsory powers. They appear to us to be entirely consistent with a substantial body of psychiatric opinion.

The decision to section

Mr Thorold argued strongly in his opening to the Inquiry that the legal impediment to readmission under the Act's criteria is in fact far less strict than psychiatrists believe. We set out his argument in full, since it will help the reader to appreciate the point:

In December 1985 Mr Justice McCullough delivered a judgment in a case involving token recalls from leave of absence under section 3, for the purpose (as the doctors saw it) of renewing their power to grant a fresh 6 months leave of absence (see *R* v. *Hallstrom ex parte W, R* v. *Morgan ex parte L*).[7] He ruled such token recalls invalid, and albeit now nearly 9 years ago, laid some of the seeds for the current debate on community supervision orders.

He concluded, after extensive argument, that 'section 3 only covers those whose mental condition is believed to require a period of in-patient treatment', and that it was not proper reason for invoking section 3 if the only treatment required was injections in the community.

Neither of the patients W or L in that case were thought to be dangerous to others, whereas in a condition of relapse Andrew Robinson certainly was. It may be that the doctors or social workers involved in Andrew Robinson's case were taking too restrictive a view of the Act and the interpretation of it in the *Hallstrom* case.

Even before relapse, when Andrew Robinson became non-compliant with medication, it could be said that he needed more than token inpatient treatment. The near certainty of imminent deterioration, combined with the consequential risks to his own health and the safety of others, the latter capable of being seriously threatened, would have been grounds enough for saying that he needed to receive medical treatment. Did it need to be 'in a hospital', the crux of the *Hallstrom* case?

[7] See above, n.2.

One could test this view by considering the state of play as at the 4 January 1993, when Andrew Robinson then declined his depot injection entirely. He had only been accepting half of the prescribed dose for the previous 2^+ months. Could it not then be said of him that he then needed *inpatient* treatment, for the following reasons:

(a) consideration of the pharmacokinetics arising would have indicated that his levels of drug had already declined below the necessary and desirable;
(b) he, at that stage, would certainly not have accepted this. Indeed, with the sedative effect of the medication lifted, but enough anti-psychotic effect enduring, he would think he was exceptionally well, and would have been highly resistant to receiving further medication. His lack of insight into the need for medication had been re-inforced;
(c) he needed to be re-stabilised on an appropriate level of medication, and finding this level once again required not merely periodic injections in the community, with weekly observations, but the much more comprehensive assessment that would only have been possible in a hospital setting;
(d) he needed to re-develop insight into his condition and then to come to terms with the need for medication, which he would be most unlikely to have done as an out-patient;
(e) since relapse could, and most probably would, generate threatening ideation, with no guarantee that it would not translate into action, the margins of safety were never great. A wait and see approach, with Andrew Robinson on the community, was risky.

By contrast, in this case, and one might say consistent with a great deal of psychiatric practice generally, both doctors and social workers seem to have felt that his mental illness needed to 'ripen' before they could intervene, however much they regarded the progression to full ripeness as inevitable. It is difficult to know whether this was seen as therapeutically desirable, or thoroughly undesirable, but forced upon doctors by the terms of the Act. It is a question that which the Committee will doubtless wish to put to both doctors and social workers at many stages in this case.

I have canvassed above an argument that it was not in fact forced by the terms of the Act, for the reason that it would have been too simplistic to formulate his needs as being for medication only, and that as soon as his needs were recognised to require care and observation involving some in-patient treatment, there is no *legal* impediment to intervention.

The Revised Code of Practice (1993), published pursuant to section 118 of the Act, says that those assessing the patient must consider any evidence suggesting that the patient's mental health will deteriorate if he does not receive treatment, and the reliability of such evidence. It also says in clear terms that risk to others can properly be taken into account.

None of this is to deny that there are thought to be difficulties under the Act in responding to the deteriorating patient. The Department of Health's current proposals for supervised discharge specifically do not include powers to require discharged patients to receive treatment, whether in the community or after conveyance to hospital as outpatients. The proposed scheme has it that if a patient does not comply with the terms of supervised discharge, the care team would reconvene to review the case and whether the patient needed to be recalled to hospital. Presumably, therefore, the uncertainties about applying section 3 would remain, being confronted at that stage. Thus they will not restore the position available under guardianship under the 1959 Act. It therefore seems all the more necessary to consider exactly what legal limitations on a 'pre-emptive strike' really exist.

We have given a great deal of thought to Mr Thorold's argument. It raises a very difficult medico-legal issue, and it is one which is squarely before us in this case. We now set out the reasons for our view that there is probably no legal impediment to the readmission of a patient like Andrew Robinson at the point of loss of insight, when he refused further medication. He fell precisely into the category of patient which the Internal Review was set up to consider, namely a patient who:

– is compulsorily admitted to hospital for treatment for mental illness;
– responds to the treatment and improves;
– is discharged into the community with a care plan;
– fails to continue to comply with the care plan, and consequently deteriorates;
– is formally re-admitted to hospital, where the whole cycle begins again.

He also manifested other characteristics which are decidedly relevant. First, when psychotic, his ideation could become chillingly violent and aggressive. The reader should refer to p. 82 of Chapter XI, where we set out an example of his written thoughts, to see exactly what we mean. Secondly, his index offence in 1978 had already demonstrated that he was capable of extremely dangerous behaviour. Finally, and this illustrates a concern of those who have opposed community treatment orders, he suffered from serious side effects from medication. He was particularly distressed by its effect on his potency. Nobody should, and we certainly do not, underestimate the distress that this caused him. But, sadly for him, he posed, and continued to pose serious risk to others when floridly psychotic, which he becomes within weeks of breaking medication.

We have indicated above our view that, even when asymptomatic, he could be said, both in a clinical and a legal sense, to be 'suffering from mental illness'. As to the *'nature or degree'* of that illness, we see no inherent difficulty in applying this concept to a condition which is asymptomatic at the time of assessment, provided there is adequate material from past history to guide the clinician. Just because an illness is asymptomatic when assessed, does not mean that it cannot have gradations of severity, or in the statutory language gradations of 'nature or degree'. The issue concerns the features of the *underlying* condition, and in the example before us there was extensive history from which to assess the severity of that condition when unmodified by drugs. The wording of the phrase is deliberately disjunctive. We are aware, however, that psychiatrists sometimes interpret the phrase conjunctively but it may be sufficient to consider the nature of the mental disorder without waiting for the development of 'degree' in its severity.

The next requirement in section 3 is that the illness must be of a nature or degree which makes it *'appropriate for him to receive medical treatment in a hospital'*, in other words requiring inpatient status. It is at this point in the analysis that many believe that the case for compulsory admission for treatment of a patient, who has only just refused medication, cannot be sustained as a matter of law.

The argument goes thus. At that moment the patient is usually well because, just as in Andrew Robinson's case, the earlier depot injections are still exerting an anti-psychotic effect. The patient is coping with life as well as before. He needs no nursing assistance to carry out his daily functions. For a while, and the period will vary from patient to patient, he will continue to be well. After a period of a few months the patient's clinicians may sense the signs of psychosis, but for a few weeks they may be reasonably confident that he will remain asymptomatic. What, it may be asked, do the clinicians wish to administer by way of treatment other than injections? If they wish only to give injections this can be given as easily in an outpatient setting as inpatient. If the patient were to be re-admitted, and be given an injection, would not the clinicians be immediately content once more to discharge him? If so, the grounds for compulsory admission are lacking. Thus, the argument goes, the clinician is compelled, by the present state of the law, to wait for the psychosis to ripen until it calls for more than nominal inpatient treatment.

We do not subscribe to this analysis in Andrew Robinson's case. It adopts far too mechanistic an approach to the clinical challenge which he presented in 1992/93. After accepting medication for over 2½ years, his refusal of medication indicated a breakdown of co-operation and trust in those treating him. Psychiatrists are familiar with the phenomenon whereby patients who stop their depot medication can experience a 'honeymoon' period in which they feel that they are exceptionally well. It can easily deceive the less experienced nurse, as it did in Andrew Robinson's case. This is precisely because the sedative effect of the medication lifts relatively speedily, but the anti-psychotic effect endures for a while, though to a steadily diminishing degree. Briefly, for perhaps a few weeks, the patient gets the best of all possible worlds, usually without understanding why. His belief that medication is no longer required is re-inforced with time, and his resistance to resumption of medication deepens. The patient comes to believe that this time, and at long last, he no longer needs medication. If past history points strongly to imminent deterioration it is an abdication of clinical responsibility to collude with the patient's analysis at this stage.

Andrew Robinson had been highly co-operative. He knew that the Guardianship Order did not carry with it a power to impose treatment. He accepted medication, so he told us, because he did not want to 'fall out' with those caring for him. Although he himself did not say so, this acceptance may not have been entirely free from fear of compulsion, of which he had quite extensive prior experience, but we do not think that it was wholly due to fear of consequences. There was a desire to co-operate, which had provided the basis for a successful period of treatment.

It is possible that prompt restoration of Guardianship might have sustained the previous dynamics of the relationship, and with it restored his full co-operation, for example, when he began to refuse half of the dose in October 1992. We certainly think that this should have been tried, given its previous success. But with passing time it became less likely that it would, for all the reasons given above. Certainly by January 1993, when he refused the entire dose, the opportunity to retrieve the situation short of compulsory admission was probably lost.

Our view is that, if restoration of Guardianship had failed, he required more than simply his next injection, given under compulsion. He needed to be 're-engaged' with the clinical team. A period of inpatient care, possibly quite brief but certainly more than 'nominal', was the only way to secure that re-engagement. Indeed, we think that merely admitting him for an injection, without much more extensive human therapeutic contact, designed to achieve understanding by him of the reasons why medication was necessary, would have been an inadequate approach, insufficient to lay the basis for a future period of co-operation.

We draw some support for the view that the law accepts this formulation of his needs as one which is proper to justify admission from a recent decision of the Court of Appeal in the case of *R* v. *Canons Park Mental Health Review Tribunal, ex parte A.*[8] There the Court considered what could constitute *'likelihood of medical treatment alleviating or preventing a deterioration of the patient's condition'*. This is a matter to which a tribunal must have regard when considering whether, in its discretion, it should discharge a patient already detained under section 3, if discharge is not actually mandated by the section 72(1)(b) criteria. Roch LJ held:

> ... the treatability test is satisfied if nursing care etc are likely to lead to an alleviation of the patient's condition in that the patient is likely to gain an insight into his problem or cease to be unco-operative in his attitude towards treatment which would potentially have a lasting benefit.

While not explicitly directed to the question of admission, we think this is a clear indication that the therapeutic objective of inducing insight or obtaining co-operation is one which the law recognises, and which would almost certainly be accepted as reasonable and proper grounds for admission as well.

Consequently, we feel that it was 'appropriate for him to receive medical treatment in a hospital', indeed, necessary that he should.

Further requirements imposed by section 3 are that inpatient treatment be *'necessary for the health or safety of the patient or for the protection of other persons'*, and that *'it cannot be provided*

---

[8] [1994] 3 WLR 630.

unless he is detained under this section'. When he refused medication he put his own health in serious jeopardy. Any delay was harmful because insight and co-operation would become progressively harder to restore. The *'protection of other persons'* was manifestly a consideration on the basis of his past history.

For a patient with his history and prognosis there is no identifiable clinical benefit in delaying restoration of medication at this stage, and powerful positive reasons for advocating swift resumption of medication. To regard a drug-holiday as in some way a vindication of his civil liberties would be to take a disturbingly short-term view.

A review by Wyatt[9] of 22 studies of the course and prognosis of schizophrenia in patients strongly supports a widely held view that the long-term course of the illness is adversely affected by breaks in medication. Early intervention and maintenance on medication during a first breakdown increases the likelihood of an improved long-term course. Furthermore, there is evidence that patients whose illness has been stabilised on medication, and who suffer a relapse when neuroleptic medication is withdrawn, have difficulty in returning to their previous level of function and may require an increased dose of neuroleptic to achieve control of the symptoms beyond that necessary in the first breakdown. Our impression is that Andrew Robinson's mental state had deteriorated over the years, and with each florid breakdown, as and when medication was withdrawn, it had become increasingly difficult for him to achieve the level of functioning that he had achieved during his stay at Broadmoor and the early Moorhaven days. The local expert in these matters, Dr Gillespie, who had clearly advised that he 'would not recommend any strategy which includes reducing or discontinuing the medication', expanded on this at the oral hearings:

> At that time there was a lot of interest in a variety of approaches to medication. One approach was micro-dosing – to go down to the lowest possible level. Another was to target medication to target symptoms, so you would have intermittent therapy. Another approach was to have drug holidays. Round about that time there was quite a lot of research into those approaches and it appears that drug holidays were the least favourable in so far as patients would relapse about three months after stopping their medication. Intermittent

[9] Wyatt, R.J. 'Neuroleptics and the natural course of schizophrenia'. *Schizophrenia Bulletin* (1991), 17, 325-49.

dosing produced some symptoms and relapse, although for most cases hospitalisation wasn't necessary. Micro-dosing produced a very similar picture.

I felt in this case the potential danger was such that I wouldn't have advised any of those. I personally wouldn't have undertaken any of those proposals.

We are aware that the long-term prognosis for a *first* episode of schizophrenia is extremely difficult to predict and, since the long-term effects of neuroleptic medication are both unpleasant and potentially harmful, that there are many patients for whom a trial of a drug-free period will be beneficial and no adverse outcome will result, especially where the patient has a life style in which he will not be subjected to excessive emotional stresses. Andrew Robinson was not in this fortunate group. In view of the risk he posed to others, and the harm done to himself by further relapses, we believe that every possible effort should have been made to ensure that his medication was continuous. We think that the current legal position did not prevent it, though professional carers genuinely believed it did. This mistaken view of the Act has all too frequently instilled a feeling of clinical impotence in the face of medical instinct, with the law cited as both inhibitor and alibi. It is time to consign this alibi to the museum of medico-legal history.

We stress that we are emphatically not suggesting that any patient who defaults on medication should promptly be placed under compulsion. Psychiatrists have to act on evidence, not hunch or suspicion. In the absence of a very clear pattern of relapse, waiting to see whether psychotic symptoms emerge may be the only possible clinical approach. The human relationship between psychiatrist and patient often requires that before invoking compulsion there should be some clear-cut incident or development – something demonstrable – to which the psychiatrist can point in later discussions with the patient.

Different patients require different indices of caution. Delay is much easier to justify if no question of safety of other persons arises. But a very high index of caution, and with it early intervention, is essential where previous history is as disturbing as it was in Andrew Robinson's case. We return to this point a little later on when we consider practice where patients are under restriction orders.

Before leaving this topic we mention two oft-cited reasons for the relatively late use of the Act. The first is poor availability of hospital admission beds, the second, patient workload. We have no reason to believe that the first applied in this case. No psychiatrist claimed lack of availability of beds to be a reason for deferring admission, our earlier review of services had not revealed this to be a problem. Psychiatrists in South Devon do, however, have large catchment areas, approximately 50 per cent above the size recommended by the Royal College of Psychiatrists. While in rural areas, the level of morbidity may be manageable for this size of catchement, a consultant or community team personnel working in an urban area, like Torquay, would be very stretched to meet the predicted need, especially if their work straddled two different clinical responsibilities.

Andrew Robinson's case is an excellent example of the target group which we believe needs far greater priority. If a policy of closer supervision in the community, and early intervention is to be effective, the Trust will need to review both the numbers of specialist professional staff, their training and the distribution of resources across the geographical area. None of the professionals complained to us of overwork, and we certainly do not think this was the main reason for the long delay before Andrew Robinson was admitted to hospital. But we do feel that it had some influence on the way in which his problems were handled in the six months before his final admission.

The European Convention on Human Rights

In the debate on community treatment orders it is sometimess suggested that requiring 'well' patients to accept medication in the community runs the risk of violating the European Convention on Human Rights, in particular Article 5,[10] which is concerned with liberty and security of person. We, therefore, turn to this issue, because it may be argued that our own interpretation of the Mental Health Act threatens to violate the Convention in much the same way.

The leading case on criteria for compulsory admission is that of *Winterwerp* v. *The Netherlands*.[11] The essential ruling in that case

[10] Article 5(1): 'Everyone has the right to liberty and security of person. No one shall be deprived of his liberty save in the following cases and in accordance with a procedure prescribed by law: ... (e) the lawful detention of ... persons of unsound mind ...'
[11] [1979] 2 EHRR 387.

was that, except in emergency cases, the individual must reliably be shown to be of unsound mind on the basis of objective medical expertise; that the mental disorder must be of a kind or degree warranting compulsory confinement; and that the validity of continued confinement depends upon the persistence of such a disorder. Subsequent cases have quoted and underlined these criteria, but they have not changed them.

Nothing in the Winterwerp principles conflicts with the approach we have adopted. The term 'person of unsound mind' is itself very broad, and the term used in the French text of the Convention, *'aliéné'*, equally carries a very broad meaning. We no more think that 'unsoundness of mind' requires active symptomatology under European law than it does under UK law. Such an interpretation certainly cannot be inferred from the language of the Convention, nor from any reported case.

In the case of *X* v. *United Kingdom*[12] the Court held that the guarantees in Article 5 of liberty and security of person were just as applicable to the recall of a restricted patient who has been conditionally discharged following imposition of a restriction order by a criminal court. It was argued by the Government that his detention was referable not to the recall but instead to the conviction which led to the imposition of the restriction order in the first place. Both the European Commission and Court rejected this contention. But on the facts of the case the Court held that compulsory admission by way of recall was justified under Article 5(1)(e) in X's case.

No other case on the legality of conditional discharge under a mental health legal code has yet come before the European Court of Human Rights. The Commission, however, has held to be inadmissible a complaint from a Swedish citizen, that a requirement to receive medical treatment as an outpatient violated the Convention (*W* v. *Sweden*).[13] The Commission held that Article 5 was inapplicable:

> The provisional discharge was accompanied by an order that the applicant should take medicine and present herself for medical control at the hospital once every second week. The Commission considers that these conditions attached to the provisional discharge

---

[12] [1981] 4 EHRR 181.
[13] App. No. 12778/87, Decisions and reports of the European Commission on Human Rights, vol. 59, pp. 158-61, Decision 9 December 1988.

were not so severe that the applicant's situation after her provisional discharge could be characterised as a deprivation of liberty.

An earlier admissibility decision of the Commission[14] had held that such a conditional discharge, also involving Swedish law, was likewise permissible under Article 8,[15] the Article concerned with respect for private and family life. The relevant part of the decision reads as follows:

> It is clear from the decision of the Discharge Council that the reason for not discharging the applicant permanently was that there were reasons to believe that the applicant would stop taking her medication if permanently discharged and that that would lead to a deterioration of her health. The decision thus pursued the aim of protecting the Applicant's 'health', which is an aim permissible under Art. 8(2). Having examined the case file and the parties' submissions, the Commision finds that the decision not to discharge the applicant permanently was 'necessary in a democratic society' for the protection of her health. It follows that this aspect of the application is manifestly ill-founded within the meaning of Art. 27(2) of the Convention.

Finally we mention the Commission's admissibility decision in *Grare* v. *France*,[16] which held that psychiatric treatment capable of having unpleasant side effects does not achieve a degree of seriousness to permit the application of Article 3[17] – the Article concerned with prevention of torture, inhuman or degrading treatment. The Commission found Grare's application manifestly ill-founded under Articles 3, 5 and 8(1).

These European cases certainly do not suggest that prompt re-intervention, when Andrew Robinson defaulted on medication, would pose any risk of violating the European Human Rights Convention. The case-law would also appear to demonstrate that

---

[14] App. No. 10801/81, [1986] 9 EHRR 269.

[15] Article 8: '1. Everyone has the right to respect for his private and family life, his home and his correspondence. 2. There shall be no interference by a public authority with the exercise of this right except such as is in accordance with the law and is necessary in a democratic society in the interests of national security, public safety or the economic well-being of the country, for the protection of disorder or crime, for the protection of health or morals, or for the protection of the rights and freedoms of others.'

[16] [1993] 15 EHRR CD100.

[17] Article 3: 'No one shall be subjected to torture or to inhuman or degrading treatment or punishment.'

provisional discharge (or a community treatment order, in UK parlance), with a requirement to take medication to prevent a deterioration of health, is most unlikely to fall foul of Convention obligations.

Restriction orders

In its submissions to us, the Trust set much store by the decision of the Mental Health Review Tribunal in 1986 to discharge Andrew Robinson's restriction order absolutely. It said:

> It is our submission that in treating Mr Robinson during this period the task of every professional was made unnecessarily and inappropriately difficult by reason of the incorrect discharge of the Restriction Order by the Mental Health Review Tribunal on 19th September 1986. In wrongly discharging Mr Robinson the Tribunal destroyed a framework whereby Mr Robinson could be required to take medication, be required to return to inpatient treatment without recourse being made to the provisions of Sections 2, 3 and 4 of the Mental Health Act and in particular to the meeting of the clinical criteria imposed by Sections and recognised by medical practitioners.

We ourselves think that the absolute discharge was a very unfortunate event, and so we accept the general thrust of this submission. But we think there are lessons to be learnt, and so propose to explore the topic of restriction orders, and practice under them, in a little more detail.

Restriction orders provide a much more drastic power than is available under sections 2, 3 or 4. Section 42(3) of the Act says that the Secretary of State:

> ... may at any time during the continuance of a restriction order in respect of a patient who has been conditionally discharged under subsection (2) above by warrant recall the patient to such hospital as may be specified in the warrant.

In the recent case of *R* v. *Home Secretary, ex parte K*,[18] a patient who had been recalled to hospital argued that his recall was unlawful, because the Home Secretary lacked any medical evidence that he was mentally ill at the time. This, it will be remembered, is a requirement under Article 5 of the European Human Rights

---

[18] [1991] QB 270.

Convention as a result of the Winterwerp and X decisions. The Court of Appeal rejected the patient's case, saying:

> It has been held by this court in *Reg.* v. *Secretary of State for the Home Department, Ex parte Brind* [1990] 2 W.L.R. 787 that where the words of an English statute are plain and unambiguous it is not open to the courts of this country to look to the Convention for assistance in their interpretation. The words of Section 42(3) are in our judgment plain and unambiguous. There is no requirement that the Secretary of State cannot by warrant recall a patient who has been conditionally discharged unless he has medical evidence that the patient is then suffering from mental disorder.

If the Home Secretary uses his power to recall without having established that the patient's condition warrants compulsory confinement, or without medical evidence, the patient will be able to claim that his rights under Article 5 of the Convention have been violated, but that will not assist him in the short term in the UK courts. The patient K subsequently applied to the European Commission on Human Rights, which found his application admissible.[19] As a result of this case the Home Secretary must undoubtedly recognise that Parliament has given him a power which is far more extensive than Convention obligations allow. We would not advocate the enactment of any law for unrestricted patients which replicated the breadth of the power that the Home Secretary has been given in section 42(3).

What the recall machinery offers is speed. Consultation is in reality with the civil servants in C3 Department of the Home Office, who are constantly available by telephone. The psychiatrist's obligation to keep C3 Department fully informed of all important clinical developments undoubtedly acts as a discipline. It probably instils in the psychiatrist a healthy sense of awareness of the issue of public safety.

We do not doubt that had Andrew Robinson's restriction order subsisted, his clinical management would have been different, probably much firmer, and without the same degree of latitude being given to him to default on medication without return to inpatient status. If the Home Office had been informed of the more alarming delusions and thought content that Andrew Robinson developed from 1986 onwards concerning Mrs A., we think that the

[19] Communiqué issued by the Secretary to the European Commission on Human Rights, 8 July 1993.

Home Office would then have regarded medication as essential, would have insisted that Andrew Robinson take medication as a condition of any discharge, and would have recalled him if he had refused medication while discharged. This would have been, from a standpoint of Home Office practice, entirely conventional management of the case.

In the absence of a restriction order, however, the clinical realities and risk factors were precisely the same. The same risk factors obtained. It may be, however, that psychiatrists find it easier to take a firm management line with a patient whenever responsibility for it can be attributed in whole or part to the distant figure of the Home Secretary. Dr Moss's desire not to appear 'heavy-handed' to his patient probably has much to do with the human dynamics of bearing sole responsibility within a clinical setting. We entirely appreciate this influence.

We also understand that to insist to a patient that serious side-effects from medication must be accepted as the price of discharge from hospital is extremely discomforting, but relatively easier if the relevant risk assessment can be attributed to the Home Secretary as 'guardian of the public safety'. Sadly, in Andrew Robinson's case, we think that this was the stark message that needed to be communicated, as it is also likely to be in the future in his case. A drug-holiday, assuming that the formidable personal price to be paid for it could be countenanced, could safely be undertaken only in a hospital, and then only with great vigilance.

We have quoted excerpts from the evidence of psychiatrists at EMC showing that there can be concern that the psychiatrist will not be able to justify admission to an Approved Social Worker or a Tribunal. Where a patient is unrestricted, the need to proceed through the machinery of a civil section requires the former, though the latter would apply for a recalled patient in any event. We should add that there was no evidence before us that psychiatrists in Torbay faced unreasonable resistance from Approved Social Workers to recommendations to apply civil sections. Again, we understand this influence, but feel that it can probably be overstated.

On the other hand, it is less easy to find an alibi in the absence of the discipline and heightened sense of awareness that the label of a restriction order, and the obligation to inform the Home Secretary, almost certainly induce. Whether a patient is under a restriction order or not, the need to protect other people must be central to the proper practice of psychiatry. It should not need the label of a restriction order to remind the doctor of this important point.

One other feature of the restriction order system deserves mention. C3 Department keeps a master set of documents on the patient, and this will usually include trial documentation. A psychiatrist whose file of medical records does not contain the original witness statements from the index offence trial will probably be able to obtain a copy from C3, if he/she asks for them. However, in Andrew Robinson's case, none of the psychiatrists at EMC appears to have sought that specific body of information from any source. It would probably have been available from C3, notwithstanding the earlier absolute discharge.

There will be comparatively few patients with Andrew Robinson's characteristics who fall outside the controls of restriction orders, though the numbers are by no means negligible. Nearly a quarter of all special hospital patients, for example, are detained under civil admission powers, and not therefore under restriction orders. But in cases of this kind, when medication is essential to control the illness, the clinical relationship must necessarily accommodate pre-emptive action when the patient becomes non-compliant. This approach is well understood by psychiatrists who regularly assume responsibility for restricted patients, and they make the necessary adjustments to their clinical relationships in those cases. We realise that the consultants at the Edith Morgan Centre who had responsibility for Andrew Robinson only rarely had patients either under restrictions or with a history of a restriction order earlier on. They will need to take full heed of the different role then required.

Community powers

It is well beyond our remit to review the subject of community treatment orders in any detail, but the task that we assumed inevitably caused us to reflect on the current state of the debate. Some of our conclusions are already apparent. We are not persuaded, for example, that the Internal Review Team analysed the existing law correctly. And we are not convinced that there is anything in the Convention which inhibits the use of community treatment schemes, particularly as envisaged by the Internal Review Team.

It may be felt that, if our analysis of compulsory powers is correct, then the need for any fundamental recasting of the law is reduced. The proposals in the Internal Review, as we see it, could only be *more* effective if our interpretation of admission powers is correct. For example, if under its scheme a patient does not comply with the agreed conditions, the key worker would, in consultation with the RMO and other members of the care team, institute an immediate review to establish what had gone wrong and propose any necessary changes to the plan. In that review, specific consideration would be given to 'whether the patient's condition had deteriorated so far as to meet the criteria for compulsory admission under the Act'. What we are suggesting is that there is no legal need to await significant deterioration.

Maintaining a balance

Our primary purpose in engaging in so much *legal* analysis has been to distinguish the legal from the clinical constraints. We hope that clinicians at the Trust, and perhaps elsewhere, will now be better able to reflect on their clinical options. If, as a result, they feel that their powers are greater than they had assumed, this does not mandate their indiscrimate use. In any event, the MHRT system exists to guard against any over-zealous flexing of psychiatric muscle. In unrestricted cases, it has to be remembered, a Tribunal always has a discretion to discharge on the merits, whether or not the statutory criteria for discharge are satisfied as such. Patients have access to legal aid for the purposes of their legal representation, and they can commission independent psychiatric reports. These checks, quite properly, are well resourced, and should not be belittled.

The danger with pendulums is they tend to swing too far. Sage heads may read our views in this Chapter and feel that, insofar as we have suggested that early intervention is permissible, this danger beckons. The guidelines from the NHS Executive that Trusts and Health Authorities should hold inquiries when homicides by patients have occurred is already producing a long line of inquiry reports, in which ours will take its place. Each strives to find mistakes which might have prevented the tragedy. There is clearly a tendency for such reports to criticise psychiatrists for not imposing tighter restraints on the assailants. The collective impact

[20] Para. 8.14 e and f, p. 30.

of such reports has created a climate in which detention of mentally disordered persons is much more readily called for.

We repeat, therefore, that Andrew Robinson's case had unusually stark features, in which probability of relapse was very high, the personal cost to Andrew himself predictably dire, and the risk of dangerous behaviour, when he was psychotic, unacceptable. It is these features, in particular, which have led us to feel that his case called for a different approach.

XIX. Risk Assessment and Management

How is it possible to expect mankind will take advice, when they will not so much as take warning?*

The risk which Andrew Robinson posed to other people during the course of his illness was naturally a major focus of our inquiry. Ominous signs of danger, obvious to parents and friends, should have led to rapid action to avert the likelihood of the index offence being repeated. They were largely ignored. His past history provided the key information on which to assess the risk and on which a safer management strategy could be built. The details of the index offence in 1978 were not fully considered in assessing his current and likely progress.

Clinical teams gave insufficient weight to the clear history of life-threatening violence and did not alter their programmes of care accordingly. Partly this was due to an insufficiently rigorous examination of records from 1978 (see Chapter V). In part, perhaps, we judge that this is because in an area such as South Devon, most patients are not seriously violent. This may explain why there was no explicit risk management strategy to assist clinicians. Possibly, too, there was some complacency in the handling of those who did pose a significant risk. We feel that if proper consideration of risk had been made at key points during Andrew Robinson's care then events would have unfolded very differently.

All risk-management strategies, whatever risks are to be assessed and minimised, comprise the same five basic components. First, there is the need to be alert and vigilant to hazard. It is simple to walk around a ward, a hospital or a community team office and identify potential physical hazards for the workforce; it is far more difficult constantly to be alert to identifying individual patients as being a potential risk. A clinical assessment of mental state which includes searching questions designed to identify potentially dangerous thoughts or actions is not yet routine, although we believe it should be.

The second step is to decide who might be harmed and how —

* Jonathan Swift, *Thoughts on Various Subjects* (1711).

and we will consider in this chapter the information which was available to the clinical team members about this in Andrew Robinson's case. The third step is to evaluate whether current arrangements adequately address the risk, and decide whether further measures need to be taken. The fourth step is to record in writing exactly what risks are thought to be present, what action has been taken and what level of risk is being accepted for an individual, bearing in mind the practical constraints, resources available and the rights of the individual to be treated in the least restrictive manner compatible with minimal risk. The fifth, and final, step is to ensure that a regular review system is established so that levels of risk can be revised in the light of more recent information.

In our consideration of what good risk management should consist, we have been greatly helped by the contributions of our expert witnesses which are published in our sister publication, *Psychiatric Patient Violence: Risk and Response.*[1] In particular, the contributions of Dr Adrian Grounds and Mr Jonathan Potts are worthy of careful attention and are drawn on here. The management of psychiatric patients who are potentially violent to others has moved away from the notion of an assessment of 'dangerousness', an inflexible concept which implies wrongly that a patient has a static and unchallenging quality of personality, towards adopting the concepts of ongoing assessment of risk and risk-management, assuming that risk will change over time and can be managed effectively.

Although these concepts are new to psychiatry, they embrace elements of familiar good psychiatric practice, such as thorough history-taking and good communication between professionals and carers.

Risk assessment and risk management strategy are becoming much more familiar concepts across health and social services, as managers attempt to devise ways of reducing financial liabilities, but the sound principles adopted by many hospitals in their attempt to manage the financial outcomes have, we regret, scarcely percolated to many psychiatric services. Surgeons and anaesthetists have embraced these concepts with more alacrity, as the spectre of medical negligence claims loom ever larger. Their potential clinical value in mental health practice is enormous, not for

[1] J.H.M. Crichton (ed.) *Psychiatric Patient Violence: Risk and Response* (1995) London: Gerald Duckworth & Co.

financial reasons but for sound clinical ones of producing better outcomes. All mental health services should now have a risk management policy.

Assessment of risk

Assessment of risk needs to be a continuing process in which the multi-disciplinary team is repeatedly reappraising a patient's risk of violence to others as the day-to-day circumstances of the patient's life unfold. Such a process is likewise important for inpatient and community settings, and is not unfamiliar to clinical teams which practise ongoing assessment of suicide risk. We were interested to note that the Trust has done a good deal of valuable training on suicide assessment, assisted by Professor Gethin Morgan from the University of Bristol, and has devised assessment approaches to suicide risk in the wake of a series of untoward incidents of self-harm, but has not hitherto adopted a risk assessment strategy of the same kind for assessing risk of harm to others. When a patient is referred for the first time, or transferred from another team, there should always be a new clinical assessment which should include an assessment of risk of violence.

Past violent behaviour is by far the best predictor of future behaviour. This is not to say that patients are incapable of change or that future violence is inevitable, but that the context in which past violence occurred is essential to understanding when the future risk is greatest. For example, it is important to know whether the violent act occurred while the patient was psychotic, or while the patient was taking illicit drugs, or was acting under the influence of alcohol. Did the violence occur in the context of the family, or a close relationship, or was it aimed at a stranger? In the case of Andrew Robinson, for example, there was a history of life-threatening violence when he was psychotic, in the context of a desired close personal relationship with a young woman. Subsequently, when unwell, he had made threats to medical staff (reported by Dr Moss) and had become obsessionally fixated with a local woman, again making violent threats, and on another occasion with a nurse at the Butler Clinic. The risk posed by Andrew Robinson could be judged to be very high, as and when he became unwell again, and either perceived himself to be in a close personal relationship with a woman, or was preoccupied with thoughts about an individual woman. It could be concluded that when he was unwell, psychiatric professionals, and particularly women, were at increased risk.

The circumstances of any past violence need to be rigorously examined. There will usually be three sources of information available: the clinical interview; information from informants and past clinical and other records.

The clinical interview

The clinical history may in itself gives clues to past violence, but by itself may be misleading. A patient will very often give accurate information about past convictions for violent offences, and clear accounts of violent behaviour, but cannot be relied upon to do so. Independent accounts of such incidents are, therefore, essential. Patients may consciously play down the seriousness of past violence or, if it occurred while under the influence of psychosis, illicit drugs or alcohol, patients may have a poor memory of events or a mistaken perception of what happened. A paranoid patient who persistently gets into fights, for example, may readily believe that they are all provoked by someone else. During a traditional mental state examination it is usual to inquire about suicidal thoughts, but routine questioning about thoughts of others are not usual. Yet such questions may reveal unexpected violent preoccupations. The clinical history is, however, only the starting point in the assessment of risk; it may alert the clinician if a history of violence has been revealed, but without information from informants and examination of past records the assessment is incomplete. Nevertheless, the mental state examination is an important starting point; the main change we advocate in the examination is that clinical assessment should *always* include a direct search for thoughts about harming others.

Information from Andrew Robinson could be misleading. This is not to suggest deliberate concealment on his part. Yet it is clear that the seriousness of past violence was significantly down-played at clinical interview. Also, many staff found him charming; his intelligent theorising was interesting; we have noted one doctor (Dr Cullen) who told us how much she enjoyed the intellectual stimulation of informal conversations with him. There is, as we have seen, a danger of staff not wanting to discover a past history of violence; it is understandably easier to engage in a superficial therapeutic relationship when such matters are not raised, and the patient's account is accepted uncritically at face value, although the relationship cannot be truly therapeutic when such vital pieces of history are left unsaid or obscure.

Informants

The violence that family and carers are exposed to is usually relatively minor, often but not always more frightening than life-threatening. Family and carers are probably exposed to much higher rates of minor assault than is currently recognised. Families may be embarrassed to confide in clinicians about violence at home; such areas require sensitive questioning. Assaults may not have caused serious injury but this does not reduce their importance for assessing future behaviour. A thorough assessment which concludes, for example, that a patient is often verbally aggressive when under the influence of alcohol, but is otherwise unlikely to pose a threat, is invaluable information in devising a good care programme and in monitoring its success.

No overt threat should ever be ignored, first because of the importance all threatening behaviour has for the overall assessment of risk, but also because even when episodes are minor ones, and the patient poses little threat to the public at large, family members and close friends may be experiencing excessive stress when subjected repeatedly to minor assaults or threats. It can be difficult judging whether or not current behaviour has serious implications for the future when you are living through such a situation with a close family member.

There are two types of apparently minor incident to which professional staff should be especially alert, since both may indicate an increased risk of serious assault. The first type is an assault which could have been life-threatening but did not result in injury, for example, when an assailant is disarmed before major harm occurs. The second type is a series of repetitive minor assaults which are gradually escalating in seriousness. It is so easy to ignore routine minor events and to habituate to a persistent pattern of incidents. It was painful to hear, repeatedly, how the concerns of the Rev. Peter and Mrs Robinson, subjected time and again to verbal and physical assaults of a stressful, frightening kind, were not heeded by psychiatric staff.

Documentary material

Past records need to be requested and examined as a matter of routine. In the case of a patient who has committed an offence, details from the case and witness statements are needed to help understand the circumstances of any violence. When a patient has a history of violent offences, it is common for there to be a mass of clinical records giving conflicting factual accounts and differing diagnoses, as was the case with Andrew Robinson. We have shown that it is insufficient to rely on discharge summaries, which in themselves may be conflicting, and from which it is impossible to judge how thorough the writer has been in their compilation. Sometimes it seems that, when the history reaches a point of overwhelming complexity, the past history is enigmatically summarised, 'see past discharge summaries', all of which contain one or two similar trite phrases meant to sum up the wisdom gleaned over many years. There is no alternative to the painstaking methodical review of past notes.

One approach we used in our Inquiry – and should, we believe, be a standard preliminary exercise for all inquiry teams undertaking such an exercise – was to compile an extended psychiatric and psycho-social summary, or chronology of the case, listing all significant events and all contacts between the patient and professionals and with independent sector services and organisations. An example of the type of chronology we have in mind, compiled by Dr Tim Exworthy after Andrew Robinson's admission to Broadmoor Hospital in 1993, is included in Appendix 2 of this report. The chronology includes extracts from witness statements, previous reports and letters, and is much more lengthy than a usual discharge summary. Most of the consultants who cared for Andrew Robinson were asked if such a summary would have been useful to them. There was unanimity that such a summary would have proved extremely helpful. With current technology it would be straightforward in complex cases to have a thorough case summary which could be updated as new information became available. Such an extended summary could be passed on to future clinical teams. In particular, for patients who have committed grave offences, details of the offence should be passed on to future clinical teams.

Management of risk

Teams with the responsibility for managing a patient's risk must be sufficiently in touch with the patient and his or her carers to be aware of, and respond to circumstances which increase risk of violence. One of the commonest circumstances is when the patient, known to become violent when psychotic, has stopped taking medication. A patient who is still subject to a restriction order, as a result of committing a grave offence in the past, may find that stopping medication in itself can justify a recall to hospital. In the case of non-restricted patients, the care team needs to be vigilant and maintain contact with the patient and his carers. A patient who is relapsing may well default on routine appointments, and teams must promptly visit and assess patients in the community and admit to hospital, if necessary. When Andrew Robinson stopped accepting his depot medication at the end of 1992 there was little action taken, although this greatly increased his risk of violence. Arrangements were made for an outpatient appointment with a consultant psychiatrist several months ahead, at a time when there was a change of consultant responsibility, but no special arrangements were made in the light of the serious potential risk that Andrew Robinson could pose.

Communication can easily break down between a patient and members of the clinical team, or between team members and carers, or between different members of the same clinical team. Furthermore, family members and other carers may see another side of a patient not seen by members of the clinical team. Information about their fears of an increasing risk of violence always needs to be taken seriously. The availability of information at the right time is crucial, and there is a major administrative task in ensuring that systems are in place which are failsafe against human forgetfulness and work overload. When there is a high risk to members of the public, or family, or other carers, there will be some occasions when confidential information must be revealed to carers or to the police. A positive duty to disclose rests uneasily with health care professionals' codes of confidentiality, but undue delay may itself increase risk and distress.

Risk has, of course, to be managed on a daily basis in the inpatient setting, but the same basic principles apply. Threats or aggressive acts, both recent and in the past history, will determine the level of nursing observation required and in what type of ward the patient is best managed. When the risk of serious violence is thought too great for a low security unit, then transfer should be facilitated to a medium secure hospital. Saying this is easy, of course; no doubt there would be few dissenters from this suggestion. We were aware, however, that general psychiatrists in South Devon did not feel that they could readily call on the skills of their colleagues in the local Regional Secure Unit because of the extreme pressure on the RSU beds from the criminal justice system. There are no other facilities available at present, and it is clear that the service has now to make serious plans for coping with the majority of violent and difficult patients within their own acute psychiatric services. We learned with satisfaction of the Trust's commitment to develop more appropriate intensive care facilities in the immediate future.

Decisions about leave of absence must, of course, include an assessment of risk made by the clinical team and we cover the provision of leave elsewhere, in Chapter XV. The level of security and observation over Andrew Robinson during his final admission should have been influenced by his past history; we have concluded that past history, and the implications that had for risk and security, was not heeded during Andrew Robinson's last admission to EMC. If all staff were aware of the risk he posed, there should have been a much higher level of vigilance, particularly in leave arrangements and searches after unauthorised leave, and also a lower threshold for admission to the intensive care area.

An essential part of an inpatient admission is the development of an after-care programme which informs the care team looking after the patient on discharge about the patient's risk to others, and includes, in the light of the hospital admission, clear plans about how risk can be minimised. An admission allows for observation in a range of social situations, and enables the team to judge how the patient responds to provocation and stress. We have mentioned earlier that if Andrew Robinson's discharge summary from the Butler Clinic had clearly spelt out the concerns raised during that admission for the safety of female members of staff, the clinical ward team at EMC might have been better forewarned about this potential risk.

XX. Principles of Care

I can't know what you know
unless you tell me
there are gashes in our understandings
of this world*

It would be absurdly naïve to suggest that there is a simple answer
to the challenges presented by people such as Andrew Robinson.
People who are plagued by a mental illness that torments them,
distorts their perception and renders them potentially very dangerous, but into which they have little or no insight, are redoubt-
able patients for health care professionals. When coupled with a
high level of intelligence, as in Andrew's case, the challenges are
hugely amplified. This is not to suggest, however, that one should
despair. Far from it, there are certain principles that underpin good
and effective practice in relation to this group of people. None of
them is magical; all of them are interdependent. All of them have
featured implicitly or explicitly elsewhere in this report, but it is
probably helpful at this point to gather them together. It should
also be borne in mind that what are being discussed here are
principles of care, not details of specific treatment regimes. Whatever treatment regime is adopted, these principles should pertain.

When working with Andrew Robinson and people like him,
perhaps one of the most difficult balances to be struck is that
between establishing and maintaining appropriate boundaries and
establishing an empathetic relationship. Looking back over all the
professionals who were involved with Andrew, we cannot fail to
observe how few managed to achieve that balance. There was
almost a seductive quality in the way in which Andrew managed
to draw in otherwise sensible and skilful practitioners to the point
that some lost sight of their own objectivity and began to view the
world through his eyes. Dr Conway's references to Andrew's 'justifiable' paranoia, resulting from his Broadmoor days, is paralleled
by Dr Cullen's accounts of her unscheduled nocturnal conversa-

---

* Adrienne Rich, *For Memory* (1981).

tions with Andrew in EMC. No doubt well-intentioned, these were replete with danger:

> ... I have often ... had conversations with Mr Robinson, as the duty doctor, when I have not been doing anything else, sitting there talking to him ... I have had these conversations in, I suppose one could call them dark corners, but you know, the lights were switched off at night and I spoke alone with Mr Robinson in some of the areas that were not supervised, discussing a lot of issues on philosophy and spiritual matters, and I have never felt threatened by him. He intellectually threatened me ...

We recognise that it is crucial for every appropriate opportunity to be taken of talking with patients, but it takes a great deal of mental agility to reframe Dr Cullen's description as good professional practice. A further example of professional laissez-faire – collusion is perhaps too strong a word – was in the evidence we heard that the diocesan exorcist, whom Andrew had invited to discuss his delusional beliefs of being possessed, with a view to having the exorcist cast out the 'responsible spirits', was apparently welcomed into the unit when Andrew clearly was very deluded and ill. The exorcism approach was not consistent with the view that Andrew's delusional ideas were part of a treatable psychiatric disorder which would respond to medication, and unlikely to assist Andrew in achieving a more realistic view of his experiences. Our view seems to have been shared by the diocesan exorcist himself. We must stress again that we believe it most important for professionals to spend time getting to know their patients and in developing genuinely warm, empathic relationships with them. Furthermore, it is important to understand the patient's view of the world; much community care breaks down because this empathic relationship is missing; sometimes all that is offered is a monthly depot injection from a 'key worker' whose contact with the patient is transient and impersonal. But good therapeutic relationships demand good, firm decision-making and objective risk assessment by the clinician. It is these qualities in the therapeutic relationship which are so easily damaged by over close identification of the therapist with the patient's personal difficulties. At the other extreme, some clinicians in South Devon had their boundaries so firmly established that developing an empathic relationship was an impossibility. Those clinicians were just as handicapped as those who had been 'seduced', since they had no way of understanding Andrew's world.

There are tools that can be employed to assist in achieving the desired balance. The foremost of these is supervision. Supervision can be seen as a pot-holer's rope. As the pot-holer/clinician descends into the difficult and unpredictable recesses, the rope is there establishing a firm connection with the surface. The rope will not stop the pot-holer hitting problems, but it provides a way of resolving them. Furthermore, if a roped pot-holer gets lost, the person at the other end of the rope notices, and can intervene rapidly.

Appropriately tied-in to a supervision system, the clinician can proceed to try to establish an empathetic relationship. With Andrew, and people like him, there is no short cut. Time must be invested in simply being with him, listening to him, talking with him, engaging in shared activity. In a community setting, if practitioners are working with caseloads in excess of thirty, to afford the required time becomes impossible. How many of us would develop a trusting relationship in which we felt valued with someone who could spare us only an hour once a fortnight? While that might be enough to sustain a well-established relationship, it is grossly inadequate in the early stages. Yet that is what we expect to achieve with people who, by the very nature of their mental illness, probably require a far higher investment of time than average relationships. If we are to address seriously the challenges of engaging the hard-to-engage patient, then we must pay attention to the design of community services. We endorse the recommendations in the Ritchie Report,[1] that caseloads of key workers working with seriously mentally ill people who are difficult to engage in services, must not be allowed to exceed a very limited number; we would estimate between eight and a dozen patients. Large unmanageable caseloads set up the clinician for failure, to the detriment of all concerned.

Once the conditions are right for developing an empathetic relationship, with all the safe-guards that supervision provides, it is important that the relationship should develop within a framework of clarity and consistency. With people for whom thought-disorder and distorted perception are significant issues, the clinician must never lose sight of the need for clarity. Discussion must be clear and unambiguous and, over important issues, should be

[1] Report of the Committee of Inquiry into the Case of Christopher Clunis (HMSO, 1994).

followed up in writing. It seldom helps to fudge the response to the predictable inquiries of 'how long will I have to be on medication?'. If the considered judgment is 'indefinitely', then that should be the response. To give an indication of future discontinuation, if that is not considered to be a real option, is dishonest, and will backfire. One day the future will be the present. When Andrew was placed on a Guardianship Order, he was told it would be for two years, at least. The two years stuck with Andrew and his first appeal against the Order came as the two-year mark was approaching. If he had been told at the outset that it was indefinite, without limit of time – and it appears he was not – he might have settled more to continued medication under supervision. Many of the clinicians who gave evidence found repugnant the idea of removing all Andrew's hope of coming off medication for the foreseeable future, but the only circumstances under which such an experiment could have been tried would have been under conditions of detention in hospital for many months while the effects of a drug-free regime were made manifest. This might well have been an unacceptably restrictive price to pay, from Andrew's point of view. We think it would have been preferable to face the unpalatable truth from the outset, so that Andrew could come to terms with the reality of his disorder and the permanent impact it was going to have on his life.

Giving clear messages is, in itself, not enough. It is vital that the same clear messages are given by all parties involved. To achieve this consistency requires close collaboration, consultation and communication. As discussed elsewhere, the most effective route toward this state is through the multi-disciplinary team. But, within a community setting, this must be broadened to embrace other agencies that are involved in establishing and maintaining the milieu within which the patient lives. This brings into question issues around confidentiality, to which there is no easy resolution. If a patient with a forensic history is placed within a community setting, who should know; who needs to know; who can help by knowing? When Andrew arranged his own accommodation, his landladies had no information about his background. That in no way adversely affected the care and support he received. Had they known in advance, it is always possible that Andrew might not have been viewed as a suitable tenant. The care team must, therefore, make careful judgments at each stage about what information is shared, with whom to ensure maximum consistency, balanced with issues of confidentiality, within which there may be a tension between safety and individual freedom.

This tension can surface in many ways. If the patient's expressed wishes coincide with what is perceived by the care team to be in his/her best interests, then that tension does not arise. The reason that Andrew and people like him present such a significant challenge is, however, that the two interests, all too frequently, are diametrically opposed. It is to this point that the boundaries, the empathy, the clarity, the consistency all lead. The task for the clinician is to understand the patient's world without substituting it for the real world; from that viewpoint, to survey the choices that are available and to find a way of presenting the choices that, from a skilled professional viewpoint, will best serve the patient in such a way that the patient will want to embrace them. The foundation of clarity and consistency provides a firm base from which to negotiate; it also allows for a fall-back position of being directive, if required.

This means that if a patient breaches conditions of an agreed contract, action that is triggered by that breach is less likely to be opposed. If, for example, it is agreed with the detained patient that he/she must not leave the unit, and if he does then he/she will be searched on return, a search so instituted will be accepted far more readily than if it is sprung on the patient. If it is not understood in advance, it is more likely to be perceived as punishment, and resented as such. Had such clarity surrounded Andrew during his last admission to EMC, he would have been unable to bring in the fatal knife.

Likewise, the absence of a clear and consistent approach to Andrew's care during his last admission, as has been commented upon elsewhere, failed to provide the structure required for his personal integration and reintegration into the community. Empathetic understanding of his world would have produced a realisation of the pressing need for organisation to rescue him from his internal chaos. Such organisation was, however, not forthcoming. Instead, his chaos was allowed to infect the functioning of the team, so that no one seemed to have any sense of the direction of his care. This leads back once again to the need for boundaries, empathy, clarity and consistency.

The challenges will continue. There is no magic in mental health work. The principles outlined above are simply a framework for practice. For those working with patients who are known to be, or to have been, dangerous, the key principle must be to retain a tight grip on the real world, while trying to understand theirs. Risk-assessment carried out through rose-tinted glasses can be fatal.

XXI. Community Care: A New Framework

Again and again I have had the satisfaction of seeing the laughable idealism of one generation evolve into the accepted commonplace of the next. But it is from the champions of the impossible rather than the slaves of the possible that evolution draws its creative force.*

Throughout this Inquiry we heard repeatedly of the serious dissatisfaction which professionals felt about the legal framework for the care of seriously mentally ill people living in the community. When Dr Moss wrote to Dr Charnaud, a colleague in Exeter, asking him to take over Andrew Robinson's care after his recent move there, he said:

> Andrew is firmly convinced that we psychiatrists do not understand the kind of telepathy by which he is afflicted, and it is one of the reasons that he gives for avoiding us. I have also noticed that he has had so much experience of the Mental Health Act that he tends to appeal before having a straightforward conversation with his consultant. I personally believe that if we had some effective form of Community Treatment Order which allowed us to give medication on a compulsory basis, this might be the most suitable form of management for him.
>
> As it is, I would not be at all surprised if he gradually breaks down again, and gradually gets himself admitted to hospital. On the other hand, I do not expect that it would do him a lot of good for him to be detained in hospital indefinitely.

In his written evidence to us, Dr Moss suggested that a modified form of Guardianship, allowing for specific medical treatment to be made obligatory, might provide a partial solution to the problems. Dr Moss, as we mentioned earlier in Chapter XII, had made a study of the use of Guardianship in South Devon and had personally been instrumental in encouraging its use for patients with long-term serious mental disorders. He advocated in his 1991 report that comprehensive care plans, including the provision of day care, education, training and so on, should be made explicit when a

---

* Lord McGregor of Durris, in his foreword to the *Selected Writings of Barbara Wootton (1897-1988)*, edited by Vera Seal and Philip Bean, Macmillan 1992.

Guardianship Order was implemented. He questioned how often the perceived need for a compulsory treatment order was the consequence of poor therapeutic relationships and lack of proper effort or care.

Dr McLaren had also expressed his views publicly, long before he took over Andrew Robinson's care. In a letter to the *Lancet*, co-authored with Dr John Cookson and published on 16 December 1989, he wrote:

> The small but significant minority of patients with severe psychoses who repeatedly refuse treatment might better be helped by a community treatment order which would permit continued treatment outside hospital and could be applied on discharge after a compulsory hospital admission.

The authors reported an audit they had conducted on 340 patients in the London Borough of Tower Hamlets, in receipt of depot medication, and their progress during the previous two years. There were a relatively small number, 11, of persistent defaulters of medication, but of these 9 suffered serious relapse which led to seriously dangerous behaviour in no less than 7.

Dr Gillespie pointed out that it was difficult, once the Restriction Order was discharged, to provide an appropriate care plan for Andrew:

> I was quite surprised he had been taken off his Restriction Order, but given that he had then given the constraints of the Mental Health Act it would be quite difficult to formulate a plan with enough teeth, really. I think the Guardianship Order which was imposed and in hindsight appears to have worked, as a result, as far as I can see, of the trust he built up with one of the key workers.

Before 1983 local authorities had been reluctant to accept patients under Guardianship Orders under the Mental Health Act 1959 because they carried unacceptably wide powers over the patient – that is to say, all those powers which a parent could exercise over his or her child. Guardianship under the Mental Health Act 1983, sensitive to the civil libertarian attitude, however, conferred only quite specific powers: to require the patient to reside in a specific place; to require the patient to *attend for* medical treatment (but not to have it imposed), occupation, education and training; and to require access to the patient to be given at the place where the person is residing, to any registered doctor, approved social worker, or other specified persons. The reluctance to use the power, however, continues.

The White Paper which preceded the 1983 Act said that Guardianship powers were needed for 'a very small number of mentally disordered people who do not require treatment in hospital, either formally or informally [but who] nevertheless need close supervision and some control in the community as a consequence of their mental disorder'. These include people who are able to cope, provided that they take their medication regularly, but who fail to do so, and those who neglect themselves to the point of seriously endangering their health (Cmnd. 8405, para. 43). The White Paper also identified the clientele for Guardianship as being essentially the same group which is now being singled out as prime (if not exclusive) candidates for the projected supervised discharge orders – that is, patients who, left to their own devices, will fail to take their medication and fall into a downward spiral of self-neglect, in precisely the manner exhibited by Andrew Robinson in the early months of 1993.

Yet, with the removal of any significant coercive power, Guardianship Orders remain woefully underused; and even when used, they are applied mostly to older patients with dementia and people with learning disabilities. As community psychiatric services have developed, the expectation that Guardianship would be deployed more frequently has not been fulfilled.

The paucity of Guardianship Orders was taken up by the House of Commons Health Committee in its report on Community Supervision Orders (Fifth report, Session 1992-1993, vol. I, para. 27). In its recent discussion paper for consultation on *Mental Health Act Guardianship* (1994), the Department of Health anticipates the enactment of supervised discharge orders, rather than contemplating the 'beefing up' or positive activation of the Guardianship power as an adequate alternative for the supervised discharge of the severely mentally disordered patient. The Department's covering letter states:

> Given the impending introduction of supervised discharge, any active steps to promote guardianship would require a distinction to be drawn between those for whom the two powers were suitable. This is clearly very difficult to achieve while supervised discharge has yet to be implemented and the way in which it will be used remains to some extent a matter of speculation.
>
> The government will therefore be monitoring the use made of

supervised discharge when that has been introduced and in doing so will consider the evidence about the relative place of the different powers, as well as views submitted in response to the present paper. It will need to take account also of broader changes resulting from the new discharge guidance and the introduction of supervision registers.

Against this background the Government will not be seeking any amendment *at this stage* in the present Mental Health Act powers of guardianship, for example to introduce a 'power to convey' a patient. The evidence that this would, in fact, encourage greater use of the powers is not clear enough to justify such a change at present; bearing in mind also that this could arguably be seen as changing the character of guardianship in a way that might make it *less* attractive to some of those who now use it. The Government intends that a power of this kind should be available for patients subject to supervised discharge, and its existence alongside the present guardianship powers may help in assessing its usefulness.

We have already said that we believe that in Andrew Robinson's case, if the Guardianship Order had been continued, there was a real possibility that Andrew would have complied with medication. Dr Moss and Mr Steer, on the other hand, believe that the Order had served its purpose, and its usefulness in achieving compliance was broadly at an end when it was removed. Whether or not this is the case, it is clear that no one felt that Guardianship provided an ideal framework for care; it was used because there was nothing else.

Alternative legal options for care in the community

What then could be put in place, which would assist those patients whose disorders are so readily treatable and yet who pose a serious risk when left untreated? The two groups of patients who are most likely to pose such risk are people with schizophrenia and related disorders, and those with recurrent manic depressive disorders. This question of how to provide satisfactory care outside the confines of hospital walls has been the subject of much debate. As early as 1957 the Royal Commission on the Law relating to Mental Illness and Mental Deficiency 1954-57[1] argued that while care outside hospital should usually be on a basis of persuasion, Guardianship could provide a framework for giving care for some, with

[1] *Report of the Royal Commission on the Law Relating to Mental Illness and Mental Deficiency 1954-1957.* (1957) HMSO, London.

mild or chronic forms of illness, that would be preferable to continued detention in hospital. The 1959 Act did not, however, embody
the Royal Commission's suggestions.

By 1978 the shift from hospital to community care was already
well established – the peak of 145,000 resident patients in 1950
had declined to 80,000[2] and already the vast majority of patients
were cared for by short-term admissions, outpatient follow-up and
a growing band of community psychiatric nurses. Having announced its intention to review the 1959 Act, the government's
Review of the Mental Health Act 1959,[3] published in 1978, devoted
a whole chapter to Guardianship and Compulsory Powers in the
Community. It rehearsed arguments for and against compulsory
Community Care Orders to which subsequent reviews have added
very little up to the present day. In the event, the 1983 Act failed
to take into account the dwindling use of existing Guardianship
Orders noted in the review. Nothing remotely resembling a community treatment order reached the statute book.

There were, however, special arrangements for some mentally
disordered offenders in the form of conditional discharge for restricted patients, broadly a continuation of previous arrangements
under the 1959 Act where treatment and specific care arrangements can be a condition of discharge. Furthermore, a court may
dictate that a patient on probation shall receive treatment in
hospital or as an outpatient, as a condition of making a probation
order. For some years after the 1983 Act came into force, however,
psychiatrists believed that there was a 'loophole' in the law, which
would give them the same powers as the 1959 Act to allow a
discharged detained patient to continue outside hospital for a
maximum of six months then, if compulsory powers were thought
necessary to maintain compliance with treatment, the patient
would be briefly readmitted to renew the order, and discharged
once more for a further six months. This 'long leash' arrangement
was declared illegal by the High Court in 1986 in *Hallstrom*.[4] This
served to revive the debate about the most suitable legal context
in which to provide care for the handful of patients in each district

[2] *Annual Report of Lunacy Commissioners and Board of Control 1850-1990*,
illustrated fig. 1, ch. 1, p. 9, in Murphy, E. *After the Asylums.* (1991) Faber and Faber,
London.

[3] Department of Health and Social Security. *Review of the Mental Health Act 1959.*
(1978) Cmnd. 7320. HMSO, London.

[4] *R. v. Hallstrom, ex parte W* [1986] QB 824.

like Andrew Robinson who are very clearly being failed by the system.

After an early proposal from the British Association of Social Workers in 1979, the Royal College of Psychiatrists made a concerted effort in 1987 to promote the idea of a community treatment order, but the powers suggested were felt to be too sweeping, mirrored too closely the existing hospital admission sections in the Act, which gave a powerful role to doctors. The idea of enforced treatment in the community – which would entail the enforced administration by injection of neuroleptic medication and little else – did not find general favour. The proposal was withdrawn. Having retreated from this battle to reconsider its strategy, another four years passed before the College made in 1993 new proposals for a community supervision order. Perhaps the most interesting difference with the 1987 proposals was the suggestion that the patient, while in hospital, and presumably quite well clinically, would consent to the order being put in place after discharge. The order also recognised the need for a designated supervisor.

The Department of Health's own internal review report, *Legal Powers on the Care of Mentally Ill People in the Community*,[5] published a few months later the same year, was ostensibly a direct response to the College's proposals, although it followed hot on the heels of two major untoward events which had made headline news and undoubtedly had an adverse impact on the public's perception of the care of the seriously mentally ill.

The Department made three main recommendations: first, existing powers under the Mental Health Act 1983 should be used more effectively, encouraging staff training and clarification of the Code of Practice, especially in the management of potentially dangerous patients; secondly, that the period of supervised leave should be increased to a year by amending section 17 of the Mental Health Act 1983; and, thirdly, that supervised discharge should be introduced applying the principles of the Care Programme Approach. The last two suggestions require legislation and have yet to be considered by Parliament.[6]

The supervised discharge proposal is essentially a revision of

[5] Department of Health. *Legal Powers in the Care of Mentally Ill People in the Community*. (1993). Report of the Internal Review.
[6] The projected legislation was foreshadowed in the Queen's Speech on 16 November 1994.

existing Guardianship Orders and still is limited by its lack of any power should a patient decide not to comply. The report states:

> If the patient did not comply with the conditions, the key worker would, in consultation with the RMO and other members of the care team, institute an immediate review to establish what had gone wrong and propose any necessary changes to the plan ... In the review, specific consideration would be given to whether a patient's condition had deteriorated so far as to meet the criteria for compulsory admission under the Act (ch. 8, 14 e, f).

Although there is no suggestion for altered criteria for admission, there is the suggestion that the procedure for readmission of supervised patients should be simplified.

The proposals would enshrine in legislation practice which should already be implemented using existing powers under the Care Programme Approach[7] which authorities are obliged to introduce in 1991. The Care Programme Approach obliges a key worker to monitor the delivery of the agreed care plan, and to take immediate action if it is not. The Department has in the past year issued further guidance,[8] which stresses yet again the Care Programme Approach and the proper assessment of risk.

A further requirement was made in February 1994 for all health authorities to ensure that mental health services establish and maintain supervision registers which identify those people with a severe mental illness who may be a significant risk to themselves or others. Further guidance on implementation was issued by the Department.[9] The register is not a statutory 'at risk' list, but is viewed as no more than a means of identifying those who should be a priority for the allocation of professional time and resources. It is at present unclear how many people are likely to be included on local registers, although it is likely there will be many more in urban than in rural areas. Andrew Robinson is a prime example of patients whose characteristics would determine an almost permanent place on the local supervision register. The effectiveness of the local 'priority' list of patients in generating rapid response care is

---

[7] *Care Programme Approach.* (1990) Health Circular (90)23/ Local Authority Social Services Letter (90)11. Department of Health, London.

[8] *Guidance on Discharge of Mentally Disordered People and their Continuing Care in the Community.* (1994) Health Service Guidelines. Department of Health, London.

[9] NHS Executive/Department of Health. *Introduction of Supervision Registers for Mentally Ill People from 1 April 1994.* (1994) Health Service Guidelines HSG (94)5.

as yet unknown, but we judge that, if Andrew Robinson had been on such a register, it might have assisted the more smooth transfer of his care from the Paignton team to the Torquay team in the early months of 1993.

The idea of a supervision register is not new. Dr John Conolly, the pre-eminent advocate for better mental health services in the nineteenth century, recommended in 1830[10] that the majority of 'the insane' should be cared for at home by 'keepers' and medical attendants outposted from the local asylum, and that 'a register of all the patients in and out of the asylum should be kept in the central establishment [asylum] of each district or county; and all persons on the Insane List should be visited by a medical officer of the asylum ... A weekly report should be made of each case'.

Regrettably, the large asylum building boom of the late nineteenth century all but killed off the notion of caring for mentally ill people at home, as admission to the asylum became the accepted method of care, and Conolly's ideas for the effective administration and coordination of care at home have remained untried for 164 years.

Reviewing Andrew Robinson's psychiatric history, we think it becomes clear that, during the period of conditional discharge under the restriction order from Broadmoor, and during the period of the Guardianship Order, the main elements of the Care Programme Approach were in place during those times he was engaged with the services. Overall he did well. One could say that during the conditional discharge years, while he was not on a local 'supervision register', he was certainly on the national Home Office equivalent for restriction order patients, with the added bonus, from the public's and his family's point of view, of being obliged to take medication as a condition of his freedom outside hospital. As we have already said, we have every reason to believe that if the obligation to accept treatment had been incorporated into the powers of Guardianship, that arrangement too would have provided a workable, if not ideal framework for care.

Flaws in the 1983 Act

When a patient defaults from treatment at present, however, no matter how the 1983 Act is modified or tinkered with, in order to

---

[10] Conolly, J. *An Inquiry concerning the Indications of Insanity.* (1830) John Taylor, for University of London Press, p. 482.

receive treatment he or she must be detained in hospital. There are, we believe, fundamental flaws in the 1983 Act's underlying philosophy which renders it obsolete today.

The first is the Act's underlying theme that care and treatment for people with mental disorder of a certain severity require hospital treatment. Furthermore, the place where care and treatment are delivered without consent, a hospital, is inseparable in the Act from a place of residence for detention; the environment in which care can be delivered is indivisibly linked with the need for specific treatment. It is clear, however, that specific treatments, for example, monthly medication, could be administered in one place, perhaps a day centre or doctor's surgery, and the person obliged to live elsewhere in a specified place such as a supervised hostel, residential home or their own home.

The second philosophical flaw is the removal of medical treatment from the social context in which care must be delivered to be therapeutic. The 1983 Act is a means of facilitating but controlling the specific health care interventions of doctors in the lives of mentally ill people. It focuses not on patients but on doctors. Successful care from the patient's point of view, however, enables him or her to lead as normal a life in the community as possible. Other aspects of care and supervision – such as a good relationship with a key worker, the provision of social and educational opportunities, a congenial place to live and adequate financial support – are prerequisites of rehabilitation. These elements are as essential for the wellbeing of a seriously mentally disordered person in the community as depot neuroleptic injections.

The radical transformation of mental health services over the past decade, from being hospital-based to community-focused, should, we believe, be reflected in legislation. The stigmatising notion that incarceration is a *necessary* precondition for effective care should now be dropped. We recognise that there will often be times when detention in a secure place is necessary in the interests of safety of the general public, and that place will frequently be a hospital, but there are many other patients who can be, and indeed often are treated satisfactorily in their own homes or in hostels, group homes or registered care homes of all kinds. Compulsory admission powers which, as we have seen in Andrew Robinson's case, are used already very sparingly, and often very late in a relapse because of the traumatic disruption to the patient's life and the disquieting sense of failure for the professional involved in the event. Compulsory admission, therefore, should surely be reserved for those patients whose conditions are unresponsive to treatment and who have a specific need for secure care. These problems of principle, inherent in the 1983 Act, affect the care of a wide range of seriously mentally disordered people, not just the small, seriously 'at risk' group to which Andrew Robinson belongs.

With these thoughts in mind, we make here some preliminary proposals which reflect our own views – initial thoughts only, as yet not fully formed and unchallenged by wider discussion and debate. We offer here the principles on which we believe a new Mental Health Act should be constructed which we believe will provide a more therapeutic framework for care, continue to control the unwarranted interventions of doctors, and yet will provide more safety and security for patients, their families and the general public.

Professor Brenda Hoggett, [now Mrs Justice Hale], recently[11] pointed out that certain principles had already been accepted by the government in the Code of Practice (revised version, 1983),[12] the Reed Report[13] on services for mentally disordered offenders, and the internal Departmental review of legal powers in the community mentioned above. The Law Commission's recent review, *Mentally Incapacitated Adults and Decision-Making: an Overview*,[14] added further key principles. Hoggett's list of principles is as follows:

1. People should be looked upon as individuals; this includes (a) having proper regard to their particular characteristics, including sex, racial and ethnic origin, religious affiliations, social and cultural background, and (b) providing them with the care and treatment which is most suitable to their individual needs, within the limits of what is available.

2. People should be treated or cared for in such a way as to

---

[11] Hoggett, B. 'Changing needs and priorities in Mental Health Law'. Paper read at joint conference of the Law Society, Institute of Psychiatry and the Mental Health Act Commission. 'The Mental Health Act 1983. Time for a Change?'. November 1993, London.

[12] Department of Health and Welsh Office: Code of Practice, Mental Health Act 1983. (1993) 2nd ed. HMSO, London.

[13] Department of Health/Home Office. (The Reed Report) *Review of Health and Social Services for Mentally Disordered Offenders and Others Requiring Similar Services*. Final Summary Report, Cm 2088 (1992). HMSO, London.

[14] Law Commission. Consultation Paper 119. (1991). London.

promote their own self-determination and personal responsibility; this means allowing them to decide for themselves unless they are unable to do so, or some form of compulsion is necessary in the interests of their own health or safety or for the protection of others.

3. Where people are unable to decide for themselves, they should still be consulted and proper consideration given to their own wishes and feelings; this means making every attempt to do what they themselves would have wished had they been able to decide.

4. Care and treatment in the community is to be preferred to care and treatment in institutions.

5. Institutional care and treatment should be provided under conditions of no greater control, segregation or security than is justified by the degree of danger presented to the people concerned or to others.

6. There should be a comprehensive multi-disciplinary approach to providing care and treatment in the community.

7. There should be proper consideration for the views of family and carers.

8. There should be proper protection for those who are unable to protect themselves against exploitation, abuse or neglect.

9. Proper procedural safeguards, taking into account the European Convention on Human Rights, must be provided whenever power is assumed over an individual.

10. The assumption of power carries with it the obligation to provide the services the individual needs.

Adopting these principles, one could devise a power for the compulsory care of mentally disordered people – and we do not rehearse again here the necessary criteria – which:

(a) Designated a place *where* the individual is required to live, for example the person's own home, hostel, nursing home, hospital etc.

(b) Confirmed that a *specific, comprehensive, care plan* had been agreed by the statutory health and local authorities responsible for providing care, which would cover, for example, income support, daily occupation, training, education, social and leisure opportunities, this care plan to be specified and agreed between the parties responsible for delivering care with fixed review times documented.

(c) Specified separately any medical, nursing or rehabilitative treatments, such as medication, behavioural therapies, or requirements for physical investigations and specified *where* such treatment would be delivered e.g. at a health centre, day hospital, outpatient clinic or inpatient ward, and named the key professional responsible for ensuring that a specific health care plan was implemented.

(d) Provided an opportunity for the patient to agree to or challenge by appeal any part of the plan and to have the care plan and specific treatment reviewed by independent professionals.

(e) Was a time-linked power with opportunities for the patient to be discharged from the order after a number of months/years.

(f) Appointed a named care manager responsible for supervising and monitoring the implementation of the plan.

We believe that the broader concept of a comprehensive care plan order, in which specific medical treatment could be given compulsorily only in the setting of a wider plan of supervision and care, would protect patients' welfare while they were receiving medication against their wishes. As we have stressed, there will be patients who need hospital admission, or secure care of some kind. But there will be many others whose needs can be met in alternative ways. The time has come to jettison an Act which neither protects the public effectively, nor provides the care which seriously mentally disordered people require to achieve a more fulfilled and happier life.

There has been a ministerial commitment to a review of mental health law 'sooner or later'. We think the review should start now.

Appendix 1

(a) Witnesses Providing Written Evidence to the Inquiry

Mrs A.
June Burrows
John Camus
Citizens Commission on Human
  Rights
Dr Moira Cullen
Anthony Dark
Steven Driscoll
James Elliott
Dr Derrick Ellis
Chief Constable John Evans
James Fellowes
Rod Furlong
Mike Gagg
Dr Patrick Gallwey
Dr Chris Gillespie
John Hansell
June Hatsell
Health and Safety at Work
  Executive
Dennis Hext
Mike Hooper

Mr J. Hopkins
Marian Ingram
Neil Lindup
Dr Stuart McLaren
Medical Defence Union
Dr William Monteiro
Dr Roger Moss
Carol Moore
Dr Richard Orr
Judge Henry Palmer
Rev Peter Robinson
Sandra Sargent
Robert Steer
Joan Stout
Iain Tulley
UNISON
Valerie Waldegrave
Andrew Williamson
Dr Jon Wride
Jackie Wright
Dr Jo Vella
Dr D. Yates

(b) Witnesses Providing Oral Evidence to the Inquiry

John Camus
Dr Gerald Conway
Dr Moira Cullen
Anthony Dark
Steven Driscoll
Dr Derrick Ellis
Mike Gagg
Dr Patrick Gallwey
Dr Christopher
  Gillespie
John Hansell

June Hatsell
Monica Hext
Mike Hooper
Mr J. Hopkins
Marian Ingram
Dr John Lambourn
Neil Lindup
Dr Stuart McLaren
Dr William Monteiro
Dr Roger Moss
Carol Moore

Dr Richard Orr
Rev. Peter Robinson
Wendy Robinson
Pam Smith
Robert Steer
Iain Tulley
Dr Edgar Udwin
Bill Warr
Dr Jon Wride
Jackie Wright
Dr Jo Vella

Appendix 2

Dr Tim Exworthy's Psychiatric Summary of Andrew Ross Robinson (8030) dob 28.1.57, dated 8 March 1994

1976/77

During his last year at school Mr Robinson became pre-occupied with the length of his nose, believing that its profile repulsed girls. 'My looks had always been remarked upon when I was younger and even when I reached the age of sixteen, which I saw as a period of decline in my looks, I often had flattering comments passed about my appearance but I knew that, from very close up, faults became apparent and as far as I could see the principal faults lay with the nose. I was frightened that from very close up girls might be disappointed with my appearance.'

January 1977

While at Lancaster University he referred himself to a plastic surgeon in London and in January had an operation on the nose. He was 'very disappointed with the results ... and was seriously depressed for many months'. It is also said that he drank heavily, could not concentrate on his work and suddenly left Lancaster University during the middle of the second term. There were also problems to do with premature ejaculation.

October 1977

Arrived at St David's College, Lampeter, Wales. Soon after arriving he met Miss B. and they were strongly attracted to one another. She seemed keen to embark on a sexual relationship but he held back because of his doubts about his ability to perform. However, he quickly 'realised I was in love with her. She seemed to embody or possess all those qualities that I had ever dreamed of in a woman – articulate, vivacious, sexually exciting ... I then began to feel jealousy, for example when I saw her talking to other men.' On the fourth day of their relationship he was persuaded to have sex with her but this was unsuccessful because of his premature ejaculation. Thereafter the relationship seems to have virtually ended and it has been estimated that he did not spend more than a total of some twenty-four hours in her company throughout the relationship. They continued to see each other briefly for the next few days but she told him that she was no longer interested in him as a sexual partner and is said to have boasted of her past conquests. It soon became evident that she had betrayed his confidence about not revealing his preoccupation with his nose because other students began to tease and publicly taunt him about the shape of his nose. He also alleges that she went to the President of the Students' Union and said that he had been making a nuisance of himself with the fourth-year girls and had been taking food from their kitchens. 'By now I was thinking about her most of the time. I had been terrified by her treatment of me. I was obsessed by her ... I used to look at her window and I could not bear the thought that she might be in bed with another bloke'.

Soon afterwards he went to a sex clinic in London to seek help but was disappointed with the results.

(1) Psychiatric Unit, West Wales General Hospital (21.11.77 – 29.11.77). Consultant: Dr H. Edwards. Status: Informal. Diagnosis: Unknown

Following an acrimonious meeting with Miss B. in which she admitted betraying his confidence, **he took a large overdose of about one hundred Paracetamol tablets plus several pints of cider and then vomited for many hours before telling someone and was admitted to the hospital.** He showed no real evidence of depression but seemed tense and talked at length about his sexual difficulties.

On his discharge he returned home where he remained tense, depressed and obsessed with Miss B. **He had a desire to smash her face in with a brick, an act which he rehearsed in the garden.**

December 1977
Again saw a plastic surgeon and a sex therapist.
Spring 1978
Upon his return to college he told his friend that Miss B. was deliberately attacking his weakness (the appearance of his nose and his sexual difficulties). **He once visited her room at night, was locked out and then cut his wrists.** Soon afterwards he was telling his friends that she was out to destroy him and began making threats about her. He was quite unable to concentrate on his work.
Easter Vacation 1978
Had a further plastic surgical operation on his nose but it was 'an absolute disaster'. 'I was horrified by the result ... He had made everything worse. It does not conform to the conventional pattern of an actor's nose. It looks horrific when the sun shines on it'.
Summer Term 1978
'I found that I was again obsessed with [Miss B.] and full of resentment ... An acute sense of humiliation and anger and animosity, although I was still infatuated with her. I wanted to hurt her. I had an extreme desire to slam a brick in her face – an intense hatred for her.' He felt extremely tense and miserable for much of the time and would ruminate constantly about the three themes which were

inter-related, namely, Miss B., sex and his nose. 'The knowledge that if I could not better myself either through overcoming my sexual difficulties or improving my appearance, then the only alternative lay in hurting her and lessening her attractiveness. By this time she had become a symbol of power and evil to me and for my security I was reduced to attacking my symbol.'

First Index Offence

From the beginning of the summer term he spoke to his friends about getting a gun and killing Miss B.; or of methods of hurting her, including maiming, and then killing himself. In early May he bought a box of cartridges and wrote a threatening letter to her. He felt that she had ruined his life and that he had a mission to punish her for the way she attacked other people's emotions. He felt she deserved any sort of punishment and at times thought she was the Devil.

3.6.78

Having drunk between four and six pints of cider he stole a shotgun from a friend's room. He fired the gun at a tree to make sure that he knew how it worked and then went to Miss B.'s room with the confused intention of 'maiming her for life' or perhaps even killing her and then killing himself. When she opened the door of her room he put the barrel of the gun to her forehead and pushed her back into her room. She grabbed the gun barrel and her screams alerted a neighbour. After a struggle, during which the gun was fired into the ceiling, he was disarmed and the police called. Miss B. suffered a small abrasion to the forehead and some accounts refer to the shotgun going off extremely close to her head.

On Remand

(2) West Wales General Hospital (5.6.78 – 3.7.78). Consultant: Dr H. Edwards. Status: Unknown. Diagnosis: Personality Disorder.

Said he had 'achieved nothing and ruined my life' but he seemed 'remarkably cheerful and lively and showed no real evidence of depression or anxiety'. After the first ten days or so and with the approach of his court appearance he began to get apprehensive. Admitted to ruminating about Miss B. Felt that she rather than himself should have been in court and that 'a great injustice is being done'. Blamed Miss B. for everything that had gone wrong with him. Dr Edwards felt that he was not suffering from a psychotic or depressive illness but that he had a grossly abnormal personality. He was extremely immature, egocentric, narcissistic and hyper-sensitive and was given to ruminating about his appearance and real or imaginary insults. Also had a mild degree of pathological jealousy associated with powerful and aggressive feelings directed both against himself and others. Felt that his behaviour towards Miss B. was a consequence of his mental disturbance. **Dr Edwards** felt that there was no formal psychiatric treatment available and suggested that the courts deal with Mr Robinson on the basis of the facts bearing in mind the seriousness of the offence.

HMP Cardiff

3.7.78

Received at HMP Cardiff. Was tearful, unstable and suicidal. He claimed that Miss B. was still persecuting him psychologically. He was treated with **Chlorpromazine**.

13.7.78

Examined by **Dr A. Capstick** for the defence. Diagnosed as suffering from schizophrenia.

29.8.78

Examined by **Dr D. Tidmarsh (Broadmoor Hospital)** at the request of **Dr Power, Senior Medical Officer, HMP Cardiff**. At interview was over-breathing and waving his arms in a manneristic fashion. Appeared both perplexed and angry and stated emphatically that once his nose was corrected all his troubles would be over. Said he was sure that Miss B.'s evil would continue and he would still like to smash her face. Sees her as a successful person who exploits the innocent and at the time of his offence felt that he had a mission to punish her and ceased to be accountable to anyone or anything. Was unable to elicit any more definite grandiose delusions, hallucinations or ideas of reference. **Opinion** – suffering from a schizophrenic illness. Recommended treatment in a Special Hospital under a hospital order with restrictions.

7.9.78

Convicted of Carrying a Firearm with Criminal Intent and Assault Occasioning Actual Bodily Harm.

(3) **Broadmoor Hospital** (26.9.78 – 15.7.81). **Consultant**: Dr Udwin. **Status**: Section 60/65 Mental Health Act 1959, the restriction being without limit of time. **Diagnosis**: Paranoid schizophrenia.

On admission was receiving **600 mg Chlorpromazine daily**. This was withdrawn for observation and he quickly became hypomanic, talking endlessly, was excitable and emotionally labile. Central delusion was the shape of his nose which he felt had affected not only his appearance and his mental state but also his bodily functioning. He produced seven or eight pages of notes regarding this. In October he was started on **Haloperidol (3 mg daily)** and he began to settle. By the end of November was showing once more emotional lability and was very worried about his sexual orientation. Throughout most of 1979 the intensity of his delusions regarding his nose abated and he became able to see his relationship with his former girlfriend in a better light and realised how disturbed his behaviour had been regarding his assault on her. Group psychotherapy was embarked upon but was not successful because of the schizophrenic disturbance. He would deliver long pseudo-philosophical monologues and produce superficial and highly mechanistic solutions for his future. His ability to concentrate returned to the point where he could carry out limited studies. In 1980 he remained calm, amenable to control and was stable on medication. The delusions regarding his nose were almost in abeyance but he had not achieved full insight into them. At no time during his admission did he show aggression or violence. It was felt that 'one can confidently predict that the likelihood of aggression unless similar circumstances arose would be entirely negligible'. In 1981 his parents were making plans to return to South Africa and at that stage it was envisaged that Mr Robinson would transfer to hospital there prior to being finally discharged into the community again. In the event he was transferred to Wonford Hospital, Exeter.

(4) Wonford Hospital, Exeter (15.7.81 – ?27.1.83). Consultant: Dr N.K. Pears. Status: Hospital order with restrictions. Diagnosis: Paranoid state.

During this admission Mr Robinson was 'friendly, somewhat lazy and understandably frustrated by his lengthy detention in hospital'. There was no sign of violence or any delusional thinking which could lead to violence. On the ward he was cooperative, took his medication regularly and related well to staff and patients. He had a sexual relationship with a manic woman whom he made pregnant. It was commented that this gave him much needed confidence on his sexual ability and that he handled the relationship well including being able to disengage himself from her. It was noted that he communicated freely on a one-to-one basis. Concerns about his nose were still present to the extent that he felt his face lacked 'harmony'. **Medication on discharge was Depixol 20 mg every four weeks, Pimozide 4 mg daily, Procyclidine 20 mg daily.**

27.1.83

Following approach to the Home Office by **Dr Pears**, was given a conditional discharge from hospital. Went to stay with his parents initially. Supervised in the community by **Dr G. Conway**, and his social worker.

1983

Mr Robinson set himself the task of writing a book about his experiences and also took up a chiropody course. He continued his relationship with Liz and in about April 1983 she had their son.

June 1983

It was reported that he was symptomless and appeared to be 'managing most competently with life in the community'. In the social worker's report in July 1983 there was some concern expressed about Mr Robinson's attitude to women. He was very fixed in the view that women can only respect someone who dominates them and this was a persistent theme in many of his conversations.

25.7.83

A letter to Broadmoor from Mrs C. (née Miss B. – victim in his index offence) in which she expressed her concern that Mr Robinson was trying to telephone her fearing that he might 'try and retaliate' and asking for advice as to her conduct should he try to approach her. **Dr Loucas, Broadmoor Hospital**, informed **Dr Conway** who re-examined Mr Robinson. He found him 'attentive, lucid and insightful with no evidence which I could uncover of any overt or indeed covert psychotic illness'. **Dr Conway** was able to satisfy his mind that there was no evidence of 'any paranoia, bitterness or even resentment towards her' or indeed that he had attempted to contact her. Throughout the rest of 1983 **Dr Conway** continued to report that there was no evidence of psychotic symptoms and that Mr Robinson appeared well and contented and was actively occupied in his correspondence course.

This situation continued into 1984.

May 1984

The community nurse remarked that Mr Robinson still had doubts about his appearance, particularly the shape of his nose, and was preoccupied about his attractiveness to women. His medication was unchanged since his discharge from hospital.

May 1984

He moved to Exeter for social and occupational reasons and his outpatient treatment was supervised by **Dr Richard Tullett, Exvale Hospital, Exeter**. As it turned out his stay in Exeter lasted only a couple of months before he moved back to Plymouth. His girlfriend had to be admitted to hospital with a relapse of her psychiatric condition.

September 1984

Secured a place on a linguistic secretary's course at Plymouth College.

October 1984

'No evidence of any psychotic process and he appears healthily motivated and stable.' **(Dr Conway)**

December 1984

Living with his parents for half the week and spending the rest of the time in a flat in Plymouth. Doing two part-time courses, one in the art of writing and one in typing. **Continues monthly injections of Depixol 20 mg**.

January 1985

Became more fixed on the shape of his nose and sought a third plastic surgeon to give him an opinion. Was advised that nothing could or should be done regarding the shape of the nose.

August 1985

'No evidence of any schizophrenic process or indeed any evidence of mental illness at interview.' **(Dr Conway)**

January 1986

Letter to **Dr Conway** from a landlady Mr Robinson was staying with in Plymouth. He handed over a knife to her and made her and several of her other lodgers listen to a tape recording of a conversation he had had with Lady Rashleigh (a neighbour of her parents who had become very involved and concerned about Mr Robinson over previous years). The content of the conversation revolved around people from his past who had 'reared their ugly heads again' and he was frightened that the past was about to repeat itself. Also mentioned that Miss B. was trying to get him convicted again. Mention was made of an appeal against his sentence.

18.2.86

Letter to Home Office from **Dr Conway**. 'Remain of the firm conviction that this man is not mentally ill as such at the present time. He is certainly not psychotic and I am quite satisfied that he in no way represents a danger to the community at large.'

10.3.86

Letter from Social Supervisor, Mr Driscoll to the Home Office, becoming more concerned about Mr Robinson. Spoke about a murder trial in Exeter where his solicitor was conducting the defence and how Mr Robinson's own thoughts were very much mixed up with that case. He believed that his solicitor was using material which he, Mr Robinson, had written about his own case. Also believed the police were following him and sounding their sirens to see how he would react.

22.4.86

Letter from **Dr Conway** to the Home Office. Mr Robinson was living on his own at his parents' home (parents in South Africa). Visited by Lady Rashleigh who found him agitated and depressed. He was troubled with delusional ideas and felt that various messages were being conveyed to him in the newspapers using some sort of code. Had stopped listening to the radio as he felt that certain broadcasts were directed towards him. Also spoke about suicide as a way of defeating his enemies.

(5) Moor Haven Hospital (25.4.86 – 25.9.86). Consultant: Dr Conway. Status: Section 3. Diagnosis: Personality disorder.

He had been off his medication for about nine months prior to the admission and in the previous three weeks his mental state had deteriorated (see above). The Section papers refer to his 'disturbed manner' and a series of telephone calls in which he threatened suicide. Had displayed physical aggression to Lady Rashleigh and freely exposed paranoid beliefs about authority and hinted at the existence of agencies that threatened his freedom. On admission he was unkempt and untidily dressed. There was no flight of ideas or pressure of speech but he did feel paranoid about the circumstances which led to his present situation feeling 'that life has nothing to offer and that in fact he had got on to a treadmill where society and psychiatrists were thinking about things to perpetuate his position' and that he is no longer in charge of his own life. Initially he was treated with Trifluoperazine and Thioridazine but that was stopped fairly soon after admission. He was kept on the ward and his mental state assessed on a long-term basis while awaiting for a Mental Health Review Tribunal regarding his restriction order. He remained well off treatment and during the course of his stay, apart from episodes of frustration which resulted in some verbal outbursts, he never offered any violence to staff or patients.

In July the police in the Isle of Wight wrote expressing their concern that Mr Robinson might be trying to contact a university friend of his who was also a prosecution witness at his trial. The police alleged that Mr Robinson had made numerous telephone calls from a public call box to at least four relatives and associates of this man.

Between 15th and 25th August he was allowed leave from the hospital to stay with family friends. This went according to plan and he returned on the date arranged. **Dr Conway**'s opinion was that Mr Robinson was a 'sensitive, rather friendless and untrusting individual' who has 'an attractive personality but who alarms people with his occasional impatience and intermittent demanding attitude and periodic restless behaviour'. The discharge summary continues 'During the course of his stay there is nothing to suggest an underlying diagnosis of paranoid schizophrenia and it became more clear that really this was a personality disorder. It also became clear that as a result of his stay in Broadmoor there was no doubt that he had become psychologically scarred by this experience and that under the circumstances **Dr Conway** felt that his paranoia was probably justified.'

17.9.86
> Section 3 rescinded.

19.9.86
> Mental Health Review Tribunal discharged him from his restriction order. Was discharged a week later to return to his parents' home and no follow-up was arranged although it was left open to him to return to the outpatient clinic if required.

21.10.86
> Letter from Mr Peter Robinson (father) to **Dr Conway**. Mr Robinson smashed a radio his mother was listening to, shouted and swore at her for listening to 'that neo-Nazi terrorist organisation, the BBC'. When his father tried to intervene Mr Robinson knocked him to the floor and attacked him 'in a very frightening manner'. **Dr Conway's** reply was that in the first instance it had to be decided whether or not he was ill and even if he was, treatment could only be given against his will if it was considered that he was a danger to himself or to other people. 'I must confess that it has always been in the past my conviction that ever since I have known him (Mr Robinson) has not been such a danger either to himself or to others.'

(6) <u>Exminster Hospital, Exeter</u> (18.11.86 – 26.11.86). <u>Consultant</u>: Dr Wallen. <u>Status</u>: ?Informal. <u>Diagnosis</u>: Personality disorder.

Had been off medication for eighteen months and since his discharge from previous admission there had been 'increasing problems'. On admission he told staff that in Broadmoor 'all inmates were mass irradiated and he was convinced that he was suffering from the effects of radiation'. Also mentioned that a thirty-five-year-old woman was inside his thoughts and influencing him. 'Quite marked paranoid ideas' were present. On the ward there were 'very aggressive outbursts when he became totally unmanageable' and he was treated for a short period with **Chlorpromazine**. Also pressurised staff to test him for radiation poisoning. After eight days he discharged himself against advice and returned to live with his parents.

(7) <u>Exminster Hospital, Exeter</u> (December 1986 – May 1987). <u>Consultant</u>: Unknown. <u>Status</u>: Section 3. <u>Diagnosis</u>: Unknown.

Admitted after assaulting his parents. Expressed the belief that a woman in the village had cast a spell on him and was using occult power to control his mind. Expressed the intention of killing this woman to rid himself of her influence. Discharged to a hostel in May 1987.

(8) <u>Edith Morgan Unit, Torquay</u> (?) 18.12.87 – (?) 7.2.88. <u>Consultant</u>: Unknown. <u>Status</u>: Section 2. <u>Diagnosis</u>: Acute schizophrenia.

Admitted after causing a disturbance in the town and making 999 calls. On admission was suspicious, guarded and irrational. Had incongruous smiling. Spoke in a pseudo intellectual way. Described telepathic forces emanating from his neighbour who he believed was a witch who controlled his actions. Also had voices in his head which he claimed were normal 'for everyone who has matured physically'. Had no insight. Treated with **Chlorpromazine 600 mg daily**. Four days after admission wrote to the Bishop (his father's boss) asking to be exorcised from the witch he claimed was inside him.

30.12.87
> Went absent without leave and the police were informed because he was felt to represent a risk to his neighbours. Returned by the police (from Exeter) the following day. Mental state largely unchanged.

5.1.88
> Started on test dose of **Modecate**.

12.1.88
> Still expressed abnormal beliefs including the delusion that he was being interfered with sexually. Claimed he was being influenced by a woman in the village and that a doctor in the hospital was capable of reading his mind. Section 2 was allowed to expire (it was argued that transferring him to Section 3 would destroy the therapeutic

alliance that had built up and could lead to a deterioration in his mental state).

7.2.88

Mental state 'fairly stable'. On **Modecate 100 mg ? weekly**. The plan was to discharge to Park View.

(9) Edith Morgan Unit, Torquay (9.5.88 – ? June 88). Consultant: Unknown. Status: Informal. Diagnosis: Schizophrenia.

By now living in a bedsit in Paignton. Believed that people could read his letters of complaint (re the system) clairvoyantly. Also believed that the postmistress in Stoke Fleming was exerting influence over him in a 'predominantly sexual way'. Said he wished to attain psychic enlightenment through a full sexual relationship but was blocked from doing this by females and the system. Mental state examination showed evidence of an inappropriate affect and a preoccupation with feelings of control. Abnormal belief that his soul was possessed by satanic forces and his spirit was damaged. Was not on medication. **The following day went absent without leave and travelled to Scotland and back where he apparently met someone whom he said could be his spirit. Returned to the ward after three days.**

24.5.88

Haldol Decanoate depot (400 mg) started.

27.5.88

Talked about being caught up by the 'system'. Said he felt psychiatrists see things differently to other people and once in their clutches they never let go. Believes that the episode leading to the present admission was due to Dr Udwin (Broadmoor Hospital) visiting him 'spiritually' and 'killing his soul, sending it to hell'.

? June

Went absent without leave.

1987/88

Up to four further admissions to the Edith Morgan Unit, Torquay. No details at present.

(14) Edith Morgan Unit, Torquay (11.11.88 – 13.2.89). Consultant: Dr Moss. Status: Section 2, later Section 3. Diagnosis: Schizophrenia.

Had exhibited threatening behaviour towards a woman (Mrs A.). Preoccupied with her, believing she represented a force of evil and was capable of influencing and controlling him through psychic powers. Been seen visiting the area on several occasions and he believed he should get rid of her in order to set his mind at rest. Was arrested after he sent a letter to her which disturbed her greatly. **One or two months beforehand Mr Robinson's landlady had notified the psychiatric team that he had**

a gun. This was handed over without difficulty and mental state examination at the time did not reveal any gross disturbance. It was felt he was probably not receiving any medication from his general practitioner. Because of concerns about his dangerousness he was referred to the forensic psychiatry service.

3.12.88

Told **Dr Moss** that he believed pillars of society were all spiritual beings and he aspired to a deeper use of psychic powers. Claimed that while in Broadmoor he collaborated with others in an attempt to expose the system. He later felt that Mrs A. was trying to obstruct this initiative. He wrote a letter with the intention of cutting off her psychic powers.

13.12.88

A letter he had written to Mrs A. was discovered by staff which indicated that his thought processes were more sinister than was apparent from his conversation and interaction on the ward.

January 1989

He was more settled but still expressing abnormal beliefs about the psychic world. Added that Mrs A. had been having fun at his expense initially in a sexual way and then more sadistic. Believed **Dr Moss** was psychic and could read his thoughts.

25.1.89

Was very disturbed and verbally aggressive. 'Almost out of control'. Anger was directed towards his consultant, psychiatrists and the system.

9.2.89

Seen by Dr Gallwey, Consultant Forensic Psychiatrist. Mr Robinson explained to him how Mrs A. looked at him in a way that he felt was sexual and how she attempted to control and influence him by magical means. Added he could hear her talk through telepathic messages and this put enormous pressure on his mind. Further assessment at the Butler Clinic recommended and was therefore transferred to the Butler Clinic RSU.

(15) Butler Clinic RSU (13.2.89 – August 1989). Consultant: Dr Gallwey. Status: Section 3. Diagnosis: Chronic Schizophrenia.

Affect was flat, at times incongruous and he displayed woolly thinking. Delusions regarding Mrs A. were present. Told staff he would make his stay worthwhile by killing someone and he threatened to kill doctors or nurses by stabbing them. However no physical violence offered. At one point he told staff that Mrs A. had died in a climbing accident – later found to be untrue and when a friend of Mr Robinson's committed suicide he claimed that Mrs A. had sent spirits to kill his friend. Typed his 'autobiography' which included much sadistic material such as 'I had to think up a torture for Mrs A. I thought I should tie her up and then approach her with a power-driven chain saw and cut off the fingers of her hands. I would feed her them to keep her alive, then I would saw off her hand for the next meal. I would go on up the arms sawing slices to keep her alive for a week.' With medication his mental state improved and paranoid thinking subsided to the extent that he did not express it. Developed an unreciprocated attachment to a female staff nurse and tried to talk to her in a disinhibited way. When confronted about this he became very threatening towards her and 'full precautions' were taken for her safety. At the end of his time at the Clinic was having unescorted community parole for up to four hours a day. Medication on discharge was **Clopixol 300 mg two weekly.**

(16) Edith Morgan Unit, Torquay (1.8.89 – 16.11.89). Consultant: Unknown. Status: Section 3. Diagnosis: Schizophrenia.

Upon return had no greater insight than before. Referred to a 'psychokinetic' link with Mrs A.

16.8.89
> **Seen by Dr Gillespie (Neuropsychiatrist?)** re side effects from medication. His impression was of Parkinsonism with early Buccomasticatory Syndrome. He queried whether there was a psychogenic cause to his impotence and advised that Mr Robinson was potentially extremely dangerous to others and cautioned against decreasing or discontinuing his neuroleptics.

29.9.89
> **Was very tense and embittered. 'I wish I had killed somebody'. Was feeling hostile to all in 'atheist small Britain and especially Dr Moss'.**

8.10.89
> **Expressing anger against Dr Moss whom he believed was 'unreasonably controlling his life'. Was angry at the proposed restrictions under the Guardianship Order.**
> Discharged on same amount of medication to live with a landlady and attend a day centre, all under the provisions of the Guardianship Order.

(17) Edith Morgan Unit, Torquay (12.4.90 – 29.6.90). Consultant: Dr Moss. Status: ?Informal. Diagnosis: Schizophrenia.

Two days beforehand he had taken an overdose of Orphenadrine (3½ g) following an argument with his mother. On admission was aggressive and uncooperative and disinhibited. It was also felt he was hallucinating. **Dose of Clopixol remained constant at 300 mg fortnightly.** At the time of discharge there were no delusions but his attitude was described as being persecutory and anti-authoritarian. He was discharged to a hostel in Paignton.

Mid-1991
> Had moved to a group home and was attending a day centre twice a week. **Medication at previous dose.**

December 1991
> **Having refused previous depot, he accepted a reduced amount (200 mg of Clopixol).**

> Throughout the first half of 1992 his mental state remained stable and he 'appeared to be doing well'.

January, February, March 1992
> 'Appears very well. Talked rationally.'

July 1992
> Was asked to leave his hostel (reasons unknown) and moved to a flat in Torquay. Guardianship Order rescinded at about this stage.

September 1992
> Frequency of depot injections reduced from two weekly to three weekly. Told an occupational therapist he had 'emerged from the tunnel of the occult'.

22.10.92
> **Accepted only half the dose of his depot.**

27.10.92
> Felt his thoughts were being guided by powers outside him.

12.11.92
> **Accepted half the depot.**

16.11.92
> No evidence of any psychotic symptoms.

January 1993
> **Refused depot altogether.** 'No longer needed a strait jacket'. He claimed to be thinking more clearly and was pleased that his libido was returning. Accepted that he had suffered from an illness but disputed the label 'at a theoretical level'.

February 1993
> Moved back to Torquay because he claimed he was being targeted as a mental health patient. Was becoming more agitated and stated that the system was out to get him. No obvious symptoms were noted but there was a general paranoid flavour to his speech. Still refusing medication.

March 1993
> Refusing supervision from community nurse or doctors. Refusing medication and 'evidently deteriorating'. Wrote a letter that was preoccupied with killing people.

9.3.93
> Visited by community key worker, consultant, social worker, general practitioner and police but refused entry.

12.3.93
> Seen by consultant. 'Psychotic but not too bad'.

22.3.93
> 'Quite disturbed' and very paranoid under the surface. Family also

agitating for his admission but this was not thought to be feasible, because of criteria for Mental Health Act, until June 1993.

(18) Edith Morgan Unit, Torquay (9.6.93 – 1.9.93). Consultant: Dr McClaren. Status: Section 3. Diagnosis: Schizophrenia.

Had been a three or four month history of decline in his health care. On admission he was guarded, agitated and there was evidence of formal thought disorder and mild persecutory delusions. It was also felt that he was not revealing underlying positive symptoms of psychosis and it was noted that he had posed a major threat to others in the past when in relapse. Inappropriate behaviour during interview was noted as well as his avoidance of whole questions designed to elicit positive symptoms.

24.6.93
Depixol was increased to 60 mg weekly.

At the end of June was expressing persecutory beliefs that people wanted to kill him and **the depot was changed to Clopixol 300 mg fortnightly.**

4.7.93
Claims he took ten Temazepam tablets and 200 mg Chlorpromazine because he could not sleep.
23.7.93
Thought disordered with loosening of association. No persecutory delusions elicited and denied voices.

Throughout August was restless and over-active but caused no management difficulties.
28.8.93
Went absent without leave from hospital. Made his way to London to deliver a statement from the Visitors' Gallery in the House of Commons. Several of his delusional ideas involved John Major, for example how he controlled twenty-seven car accidents a day, how Mr Robinson's soul had been partially destroyed by John Major etc. Numerous typed notes were found in his flat and in his jacket making reference to John Major. House of Commons in recess so he returned to the hospital on 31st August. On his return his mental state was re-examined. He was found to be dishevelled, unkempt, agitated and excited. He was 'paranoid'. Had disjointed speech and was probably thought disordered.
1.9.93
The following day he telephoned his father asking for the manuscript called 'Victim of the Magic Circle' that he (Mr Robinson junior) had written. His father said he could not find it and Mr Robinson blamed John Major for taking it. In his interview with the police Mr Robinson

refers to being 'frustrated' because his father could not find the manuscript. To Mr Robinson this manuscript was extremely important. 'It was my whole life, my whole soul.' He added 'I felt I had to act then because the situation was desperate'.

Second Index Offence – 1 September 1993

It is alleged that Mr Robinson entered the bedroom where Georgina Robinson, an occupational therapist (no relation), was talking to a second patient. Mr Robinson approached her and stabbed her several times in the upper chest and neck with a knife. Members of medical and nursing staff alerted by the screams of the second patient. When they arrived in the room Mr Robinson was standing with his hands by his side looking down at the victim on the floor. The knife was also on the floor. He is alleged to have said 'I'm sorry it was her. I meant it for Dr Monteiro.' In his interview with the police Mr Robinson refers to his belief that the only way to escape his problem which involved psychiatry was to take a drastic course of action. He referred to the victim as being the symbol of psychiatry (although he had mistakenly thought that she was a nurse). 'I'd be able to escape psychiatry, it would be my route out of psychiatry. I did not know I wanted to (kill her), I wanted to make a real protest.' Arrested by the police at the scene and charged with the attempted murder of the occupational therapist. She subsequently died of her injuries five weeks later and he was re-charged with her murder.

Custody

HMP Exeter

3.9.93
Received into Exeter Prison. Appeared 'Calm and fairly well controlled'. Told staff he had been writing for some years 'about the organisation of the universe'.
8.9.93
Transferred to HMP Bristol.

HMP Bristol

8.9.93
Received from HMP Exeter. Staff overheard him say to other prisoners that he could 'rip the throat out of any doctor or staff when he gets the chance'. The following day he told staff he had been released from Broadmoor ten years previously but they would not let him go completely. Expressing paranoid ideas about politicians and psychiatrists. **Refused all anti-psychotic medication.** Was disinhibited, openly masturbating in his cell – and on occasions seemed to talk to himself. Spent much of the time either writing or walking

around his cell. Referred to Broadmoor Hospital for Special Hospital opinion.

7.10.93

Seen by **Dr T. Exworthy, Senior Registrar, Broadmoor Hospital** in Bristol Prison. Refused to enter the office where Dr Exworthy was waiting and the interview had to be conducted through the wicket in the cell door. Throughout the interview he was extremely restless, had intense eye contact and a broad grin for much of the time. Delusions of persecution prominent. Saw himself as being in conflict with 'the system' and was referring to authority in general and psychiatry and politicians in particular. Also marked degree of grandiosity to his presentation claiming that he had 'everything there is to say about true wisdom'. Also said he had written eight books on the mind, wisdom and the occult and before writing a book on the cure of madness he had to understand madness and the system and to work through the whole of the occult. There was a mild degree of formal thought disorder. Denied auditory hallucinations and had no insight into his condition. Felt unfit to plead. **Opinion**: Presentation and current mental state consistent with a relapse of schizophrenia. Requires inpatient treatment and because of the grave danger he represents to others and in particular women treatment should take place in a maximum security hospital.

28.10.93

Admitted to Broadmoor Hospital under Section 48/49 of the Mental Health Act 1983.

Dr T. Exworthy
Senior Registrar to Dr D. Mawson
8 March 1994

Appendix 3

Statement of the Committee of Inquiry into the Circumstances Leading up to and Surrounding the Fatal Incident at the Edith Morgan Centre on 1st September 1993, made at the Preliminary Hearing at Torbay Hospital, 16th May 1994 at 12 Noon

The Committee's Terms of Reference are:

> To inquire into the circumstances leading up to, and surrounding the admission of Andrew Robinson to the Edith Morgan Centre, Torbay; and the incident on 1 September 1993 in which he fatally assaulted Georgina Robinson, who subsequently died on 7 October 1993; and to consider the lessons and implications arising with a view to making suitable recommendations.

The Committee has already indicated that, to the extent only that the inquiry will involve an examination of the routine at the Centre in permitting patients freedom of movement in and out of the Centre (including the use of the power under Section 17, Mental Health Act 1983 by Responsible Medical Officers to grant leave of absence) it will take evidence about the circumstances of the suicide of Stephen Hext in Torquay on 15 December 1993, and any other similar cases.

The Committee repeats herewith the three distinct parts into which its Inquiry will fall:

(1) To investigate what actually happened on 1 September 1993 when the incident at the Edith Morgan Centre took place.

(2) To investigate (i) Andrew Robinson's clinical history, so far as known and relevant to the matters under review; and (ii) his involvement with mental health services, in particular, services in the Torbay area during the period leading up to his admission to the Edith Morgan Centre.

(3) To consider the lessons and implications arising, with a view to making recommendations. This is likely to include consideration of the following matters:

    (a) the influences of architectural factors, and the possible modification to the Edith Morgan Centre itself, and to the client group admitted and treated there;

    (b) the state of the art of the assessment of risk and prediction of dangerousness posed by patients;

    (c) the control and discipline of psychiatric patients – in particular, how incidents caused by patients are managed by staff;

    (d) the availability of hospital beds in other facilities, such as the

Butler Clinic, or the special hospital system, so far as this affects the sound management of the Edith Morgan Centre.

In 1993, after the tragic incident, but before the death of Miss Robinson and before the establishment of this Inquiry, the same three members of the Committee of Inquiry were asked by the Chairman of the South Devon Healthcare Trust, Mr Anthony Boyce, 'To study and report on the mental health care in South Devon, with special reference to the general acute services; and to make recommendations'. Its report was published on 18 April 1994. (Copies will be available at the Preliminary Hearing on 16 May 1994.)

While that Review had different terms of reference, there has inevitably been some overlap with the scope of the present Inquiry. The Committee thinks it helpful to refer to some of the specific recommendations which touch on the Committee of Inquiry's terms of reference.

In our <u>Recommendation 23</u> we said that:
(a) The Edith Morgan Centre, unmodified, is seriously prejudicial to effective mental health care, and should rapidly undergo plans for modification;
(b) Such plans should be drawn up by a small working-group under the direction of a project officer.

In our <u>Recommendation 24</u> the Committee urged that planning should start on the re-provision of in-patient facilities away from the site of the District General Hospital.

In our <u>Recommendation 26</u> the Committee urged that a strategy be devised and aimed at promoting the safety and security of patients, staff and the public and that it should include (inter alia) mechanisms for informing staff of individual patients' propensities to violence, and incident reporting system.

These recommendations are, the Committee thinks, uncontroversial; they were widely supported by those who gave evidence to the Committee. Anybody who would wish to take issue with the analysis in the report, so far as it touches on our terms of reference for the present Inquiry, should nevertheless feel entirely free to do so. Any queries about the Inquiry should be made to the secretary to the Inquiry, Ms Penny Allsop, who can be contacted at the Headquarters of the South Devon Healthcare Trust.

The Committee has already invited anybody who possesses information about the subject matter of the Inquiry to provide his/her evidence in writing, such matter to be submitted not later than 30 June 1994. The Committee may, in addition, interview witnesses whom it regards as able to supply relevant information; and statements will be taken for the sole purpose of the Inquiry. The Committee will decide whom it will ask to come and give evidence at the oral hearings to be held in the Long Room, Old Forde House, Brunel Road, Newton Abbot on 18, 19, 20, 21, 25, 26, 27 and

28 July 1994 and such other days thereafter as may be deemed necessary.
It will give such witnesses ample notice of the precise date and time of
attendance.

The Committee is intending, well in advance of the oral hearings, to
supply an analysis of the psychiatric record of Andrew Robinson, which
should materially assist those wishing to give evidence to the Inquiry.
Indeed, the Committee would be grateful if potential witnesses could
supply any additional material which would lead to the compilation of a
complete psychological and psychiatric profile of Andrew Robinson. This
document would be available to all the parties at the oral hearings and
thus obviate such investigation of facts which would otherwise have to be
canvassed.

The Committee intends further to conduct, at the conclusion of the oral
hearings – it is hoped, on 1 and 2 August 1994 – two seminars at which
key figures in the mental health system will be asked to engage in a
dialogue with the Committee and the parties to the Inquiry on two issues.
First, the appraisal and assessment of patient violence; and, secondly,
institutional and individual responses to inpatient violence. Information
about the guest-speaker participants to the seminar will be supplied in the
course of the next few weeks.

The Committee wishes at the outset of the Inquiry to stress that this is
an Inquiry. It is distinctly not a piece of litigation familiar to English
lawyers, with rival contentions being disputed in a legal form. All decisions
about the procedure for the conduct of the Inquiry will be taken now by
the Committee, subject to any submissions that may be made at the end
of this statement. The Committee will at the same time entertain applications for legal representation, granted strictly on the basis that the party
needs to protect some right or interest which may be thought reasonably
to be in jeopardy or subject to potential criticism. Any legal representation
which is granted can be only at the expense of that party. Such legal
representation is intended primarily to assist the Committee in its inquiry;
only secondarily is the legal representative empowered to promote the
cause of his/her client.

A number of consequences flow from this functioning of legal representation. First, the Committee alone will decide who is to be invited to
give oral evidence, although if there is any request for someone to be called
as a witness, the Committee will consider such request. Notice will be given
in advance of a witness being called to give evidence.

The Committee will decide to what matters any evidence shall be directed. In advance of witnesses being called to give evidence, they will be
required to give the secretariat to the Committee a written statement, if
such statement has not already been supplied to the Committee. All
written statements will be made available to the parties as much in
advance of the witness giving evidence as is possible.

There is no right in any party before the Inquiry asking questions of any
witness. Nevertheless, the Committee proposes to allow questions to be
asked, but only to the extent that the Committee considers that it will
positively assist in eliciting useful information. Questioning will be se-

verely restricted to matters related to the events and conduct of persons involved in the subject matter of the Inquiry. The Committee will exercise control in all questioning. The parties are warned that any unnecessary questioning, in content or in length, will be prevented.

The Committee expects shortly to have gathered all relevant documentation from the relevant sources, and will be making the documentation available to the parties in advance of the oral hearings. If anybody has in his/her possession any relevant documents, the Committee would be grateful if they were supplied. The originals will be retained throughout the Inquiry, but returned to their owner after the Committee has ceased to have use of them.

Subject to any submission made at the conclusion of this statement, the Committee intends to conduct its oral hearings in public. That means that the media are entitled to cover the hearings, contemporaneously or retrospectively, by the use of electronic devices which do not obtrude onto the proceedings such as to distract witnesses and others present in the Committee Room. If any representatives of the media require special facilities for coverage of the oral hearings, applications should be made to the secretariat to the Committee.

Appendix 4

(a) Edith Morgan Centre: first floor

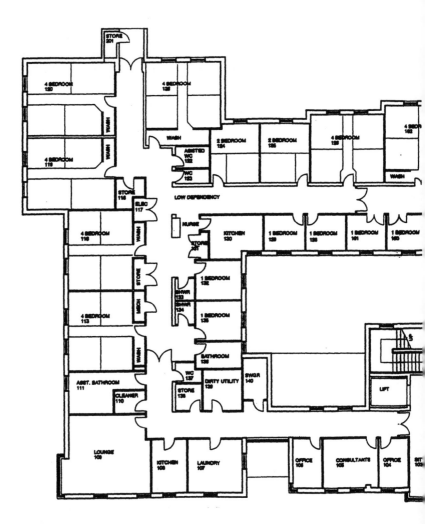

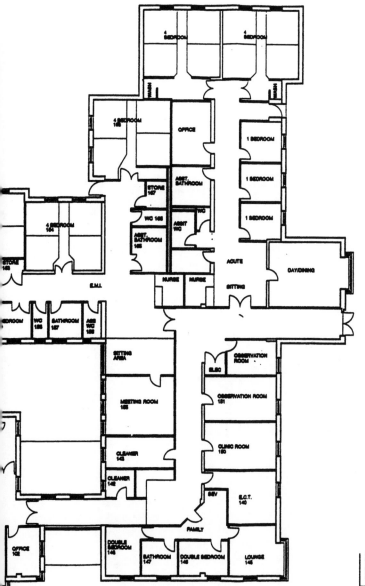

(b) Edith Morgan Centre: ground floor

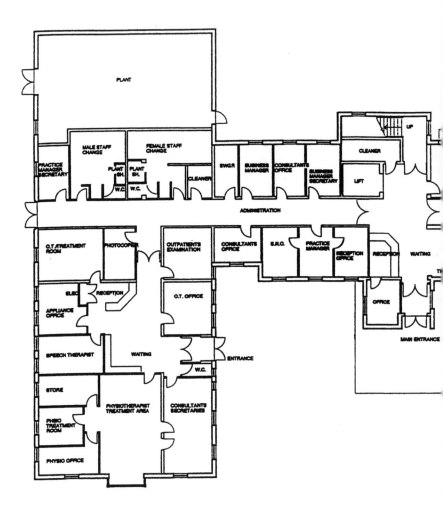

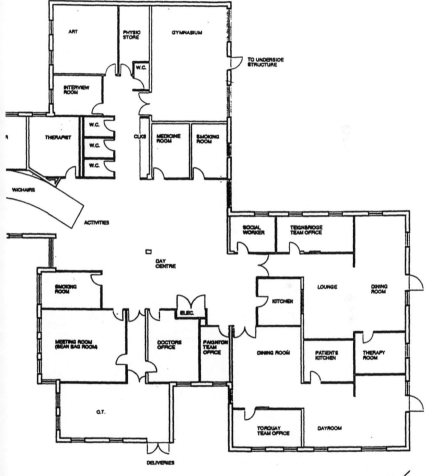

(c) South Devon Health Trust Area

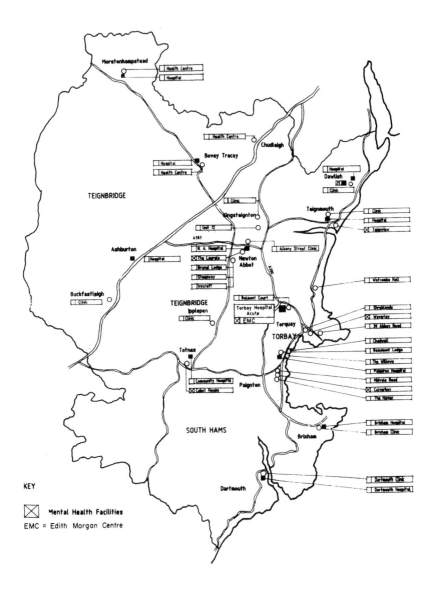

KEY

Mental Health Facilities

EMC = Edith Morgan Centre

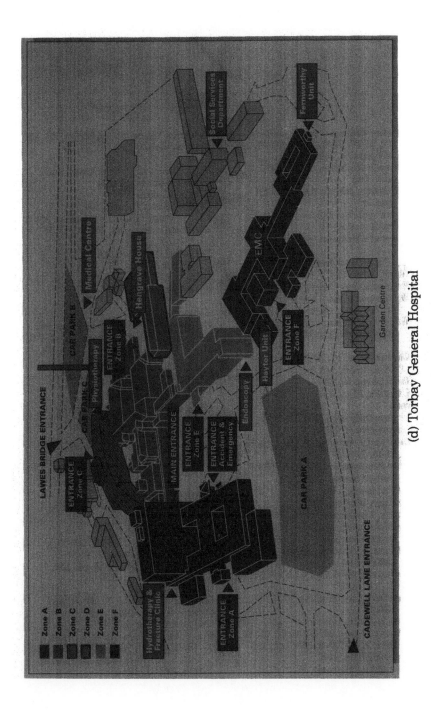

(d) Torbay General Hospital

Index